In Clinical Practice

Taking a practical approach to clinical medicine, this series of smaller reference books is designed for the trainee physician, primary care physician, nurse practitioner and other general medical professionals to understand each topic covered. The coverage is comprehensive but concise and is designed to act as a primary reference tool for subjects across the field of medicine.

More information about this series at http://www.springer. com/series/13483

A. Sahib El-Radhi

Avoiding Misdiagnosis in Pediatric Practice

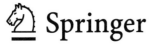 Springer

A. Sahib El-Radhi
Chelsfield Park Hospital, Paediatrics
University of London
Orpington
UK

ISSN 2199-6652   ISSN 2199-6660   (electronic)
In Clinical Practice
ISBN 978-3-030-41749-9   ISBN 978-3-030-41750-5   (eBook)
https://doi.org/10.1007/978-3-030-41750-5

This Springer imprint is published by the registered company Springer Nature Switzerland AG
The registered company address is: Gewerbestrasse 11, 6330 Cham, Switzerland

Preface

Medical professionals do their work to make people well by the process of healing their injuries, managing and curing illnesses, with the aim of prolonging life. Diagnosis indicates identification of the nature of a particular complaint that can be reached by evaluating the patient history and performing physical examination in order to find out what is wrong with an ill person. Reaching a correct diagnosis is one of the most important tasks performed by medical professionals.

Diagnostic errors may be defined as a failure to establish an accurate and timely explanation of the patient's health problem or a failure to communicate that explanation to the patient. These errors are a major concern for both patients and physicians. Patients often perceive a diagnostic error as their primary concern when they see their doctor. To support their perception, surveys have consistently found that physicians perform diagnostic errors at least once a month. When they make a mistake, the consequences to the patient can be fatal. A missed or delayed diagnosis means that the patient can suffer a negative impact on their health that leads to a delay of necessary treatment. Patients may suffer side effects and serious problems due to the treatment for the incorrect diagnosis resulting in a sicker patient instead of making them well. This can cause a period of prolonged illness, missed school or work, frequent visits to doctors, and occasionally severe health complications. Diagnostic errors contribute to a substantial percentage of repeated visits to healthcare sites and occasionally to patient deaths.

There are multiple causes of diagnostic errors. Although a diagnostic error may occur when symptoms and signs of a particular disease are atypical, masked, or absent, these errors are largely related to cognitive and system-related factors. Cognitive errors are often the top-ranking contributing factor to diagnostic errors, with, for example, incomplete taking history and performing physical examination, inadequate clinical reasoning, and unskillfulness. These are considered to be the principle causes of cognitive errors. System-related errors include instances in which technical or organizational factors impede the establishment of a correct diagnosis; examples are the unavailability of certain diagnostic equipment and the mislabelling or mishandling of a diagnostic specimen leading to an erroneous result. Inadequate staff levels and excessive workload are other important system-related factors. In some circumstances, diagnosis is obscured due to the patient being intentionally uncooperative with the evaluation of the complaint.

Although diagnostic errors are a major problem in healthcare, there are few medical school curricula that focus on these errors and how to improve the diagnostic process in order to decrease them. This subject is rarely taught to students and junior medical professionals. There is no effective strategy to teach students and junior doctors about diagnostic errors and diagnostic safety. While most pediatric books focus on diagnosis and management of diseases, there is a paucity in the literature on diagnostic errors and how to avoid them. This book aims at improving diagnostic accuracy and avoiding diagnostic errors.

Although every medical professional, even using a good standard of care, can sometimes make a misdiagnosis, this can cause harm to the patient that can result in medical negligence. Patients may suffer the effects of an erroneous or delayed diagnosis as time passes without receiving the correct treatment. A critical eye will examine whether the doctor's mistake was a reasonable one and whether under similar circumstances another professional would have made the same mistake. Those doctors who cause the patient harm would expect being litigated for negligence. Another reason for misdiagnosis is false test results due to either human error or equipment failure.

As there are multiple causes for diagnostic errors, solutions aiming at decreasing diagnostic errors are also multifactorial. Improving cognitive skills by improving professional education and training, increasing staffing levels, and decreasing workload can significantly help the situation. Increased access to specific literature dealing with diagnostic errors and the availability of consultants and medical professionals are highly ranked system-based solution to diagnostic error. Effective teamwork in the diagnostic process among health care professionals should be facilitated. Diagnostic errors need to be listed, reported, analyzed, and solutions and recommendations made among the team involved. Innovative health technologies should be increasingly utilized to support patients and healthcare professionals with the aim to reduce medical errors including missed or delayed diagnosis.

Using an extensive literature search coupled with the author's long experience in pediatrics, almost all common pediatric diagnoses with potential for serious consequences to the child's well-being have been identified and included in this book. Diagnostic criteria of each common pediatric illness have been highlighted. Adhering to these criteria is a strong argument to avoid incorrect diagnosis. Furthermore, laboratory investigation is provided to help healthcare professionals reaching a specific diagnosis among enlisted multiple differential diagnosis.

In conclusion, misdiagnosis of pediatric diseases by medical professionals usually results in late diagnosis and late start of treatment, which may have significant adverse consequences and short- and long-term outcomes on the child's health. While an early detection of a serious condition should make a difference to the child's morbidity and mortality. In this book, each enlisted symptom is followed by numerous common and rare differential diagnosis, which should be considered carefully when a child presents with a complaint. Some of these symptoms are confusing with other medical conditions; therefore, misdiagnosis can occur easily. The reasons for such misdiagnosis are clearly listed in the book, and these are followed by a short discussion of conditions causing the misdiagnosis. Our aim of writing this book is to help pediatricians and general practitioners to reach the correct diagnosis quickly and easily, and how to avoid delaying actual diagnosis so that appropriate treatment can be rapidly initiated to make the child well.

Orpington, UK   A. Sahib El-Radhi

Contents

Introduction

Diagnosis indicates identification of the nature of a particular complaint by evaluating the patient history and performing examination in order to find out what is wrong with an ill person. It is one of the most important tasks performed by medical professionals. Medical professionals do their work to make people well by the process of healing their injuries, managing and curing illness, with the aim of prolonging life.

Diagnostic errors may be defined as a failure to establish an accurate and timely explanation of the patient's health problem, or a failure to communicate that explanation to the patient. These errors are a major concern for both patients and physicians. Patients often perceive a diagnostic error as their primary concern when they see their doctor. Surveys have consistently found that physicians perform diagnostic errors at least once a month. When they make a mistake, the consequences to the patient can be fatal. A missed or delayed diagnosis means that the patient can suffer a negative impact on their health that leads to a delay of necessary treatment. Patients may suffer side effects and serious problems due to the treatment for the incorrect diagnosis resulting in a sicker patient instead of making them well. This can cause a period of prolonged illness, missed school or work, frequent visits to doctors, and occasionally severe health complications or even death. Diagnostic errors contribute to a substantial percentage of patient deaths.

There are multiple causes of diagnostic errors. Although a diagnostic error may occur when symptoms and signs of a disease are atypical, masked, or absent, these errors are largely related to cognitive and system-related factors. Cognitive errors are often the top-ranking contributing factor to diagnostic errors, with incomplete history and examination, inadequate clinical reasoning, and unskillfulness considered to be the principal cognitive errors. System-related errors include instances in which technical or organizational factors impede the establishment of a correct diagnosis; examples are the unavailability of certain diagnostic equipment and the mislabeling or mishandling of a diagnostic specimen leading to an erroneous result. Inadequate staff levels and excessive workload are other important system-related factors. In some circumstances, diagnosis is obscured due to the patient being intentionally uncooperative with the evaluation of the complaint.

Although every medical professional, even using a good standard of care, can sometimes make a misdiagnosis, this can cause the patient harm and can result in medical negligence. Patients may suffer the effects of an erroneous or delayed diagnosis as time passes without receiving the correct treatment. This may make the patients sicker instead of making them better. A critical eye will examine whether the doctor's mistake was a reasonable one and whether under similar circumstances another professional would have made the same mistake. Those doctors who cause the patient harm would expect being litigated for negligence. Another reason for misdiagnosis is false test results due to either human error or equipment failure.

As there are multiple causes for diagnostic errors, solutions aiming at decreasing diagnostic errors are also multifactorial. Improving cognitive skills by improving professional education and training, increasing staffing levels, and decreasing workload can significantly help the situation. Increased access to and availability of consultant and medical professionals is highly ranked system-based solution to diagnostic error. Effective teamwork in the diagnostic process among health care professionals should be facilitated. Diagnostic errors need to be listed, reported, analyzed, and solutions and recommendation made among the team involved. Innovative health technologies should be increasingly utilized to support patients and health care professionals with the aim to reduce medical errors including missed or delayed diagnosis.

Although diagnostic errors are a major problem in healthcare, there are few medical school curricula that focus on misdiagnosis and how to improve the diagnostic process in order to decrease diagnostic errors. An effective strategy to teach students and junior doctors about diagnostic errors and diagnostic safety has not been established. While most pediatric books focus on diagnosis and management of diseases, there is a paucity of literature on diagnostic errors. This subject is rarely taught to students and junior medical professionals.

Using an extensive literature search and the author's long experience in pediatrics, almost all common pediatric diagnoses with potential for serious consequences if missed or delayed have been identified and included in this book. The reasons for the diagnostic errors are discussed followed by a brief diagnostic criteria of these diagnoses where errors in the diagnostic process occurred. Adhering to these criteria should be considered a strong argument to avoid incorrect diagnosis. Furthermore, laboratory investigation is provided to help health care professionals confirm a specific diagnosis among enlisted differential diagnosis.

Misdiagnosis of pediatric diseases, on the one hand, usually results in late diagnosis and late start of treatment, which may have significant adverse consequences, and short- and long-term outcomes on the child's health. On the other hand, early detection of a serious condition could make a difference to the child's morbidity and mortality. Each enlisted symptom in this book is followed by numerous common and rare differential diagnosis which should be considered carefully when a child present with a specific symptom. Some of these symptoms are confused with other conditions, therefore misdiagnosis can easily occur. The reasons for such misdiagnosis are then mentioned to be followed by a short discussion of these conditions. Our aim of writing this book is to help general pediatricians and practitioners to reach the correct diagnosis quickly and easily to avoid delaying actual diagnosis and treatment.

Chapter 1
The Upper Respiratory Tract

1.1 Coryzal Symptoms/Sore Throat/Tonsillitis

Introduction/Core Messages

- A viral upper respiratory tract infection (URTI) is the most common childhood infection and the leading cause of hospitalisation and paediatric consultations. Although URTI is mostly mild and self-limiting, secondary infections such as sinusitis, otitis media, and even pneumonia may occur.
- Pharyngo-tonsillitis is defined as an acute inflammation of the pharynx and tonsils. The most common cause of pharyngo-tonsillitis in young children is a viral infection occurring as part of an URTI. It peaks at the age of 2–5 years, with a rate of 6–8 infections a year, which is considered to be within a "normal" range. Higher incidence occurs in those who attend nursery and whose siblings attend nursery or school.
- The most important bacterial pathogens are group A streptococci (GAS) estimated to affect over 500 million/year worldwide. Although laboratory diagnosis for acute pharyngo-tonsillitis is available, this is usually not performed or required in paediatric practice.

© Springer Nature Switzerland AG 2021

A. S. El-Radhi, *Avoiding Misdiagnosis in Pediatric Practice*, In Clinical Practice, https://doi.org/10.1007/978-3-030-41750-5_1

- Indications for tonsillectomy should be strict as tonsils contain T- and B-lymphocytes and macrophages and so serving the immune defence.
- The diagnosis of pharyngo-tonsillitis is clinical but often it is hard to distinguish viral (present in about 80–90% of cases) from bacterial infection. In addition, causes of unilateral "tonsillitis" are often not considered, and neither are non-infectious causes of pharyngo-tonsillitis.

Differential Diagnosis

Common	Rare
Viral pharyngo-tonsillitis	Scarlet fever
Bacterial tonsillitis	Retropharyngeal abscess
Herpetic Gingivostomatitis	Herpangina
Mononucleosis	Peri-tonsillar abscess
Kawasaki Disease	PFAPA

Misdiagnosis is due to:

1st mistake: failing to distinguish bacterial from viral pharyngo-tonsillitis.

2nd mistake: failing to consider other infections affecting the pharyngo-tonsillar area.

3rd mistake: failing to identify causes of unilateral tonsillitis.

4th mistake: failing to identify non-infectious underlying causes of pharyngo-tonsillitis.

1. Bacterial Versus Viral Pharyngo-Tonsillitis

Signs and symptoms of a viral and bacterial pharyngo-tonsillitis (commonly Group A Streptococcus = GAS) overlap. Therefore, GAS needs to be excluded clinically and, if required, by appropriate tests (Table 1.1) so that appropriate antibiotic (penicillin) is administered to avoid complications such as rheumatic fever.

TABLE 1.1 Differential diagnosis of bacterial and viral pharyngo-tonsillitis

Features that favour bacterial cause of sore throat (15–20% of cases)

- Unwell-looking child, 5–15 years of age, with a complaint of sore throat, and high fever >38.5 °C

- Tonsillar enlargement with diffuse redness and pus on pharynx and tonsillar pillars, with petechial spots on the soft palate, often with deviation of the uvula. The presence of exudate on the tonsils is the most useful finding favouring bacterial infection

- Enlarged and tender anterior lymphnodes

- The presence of systemic symptoms such as abdominal pain and headaches

- Absence of URTI symptoms (no runny nose, cough, or conjunctivitis)

- Diagnosis for GAS: Rapid antigen test has high specificity and sensitivity close to 95% and is fast (10 min). Other tests include throat swab culture, FBC for WBC and CRP. An ASO titre with fourfold increase in 1–2 weeks is diagnostic for GAS. PCR-based tests are now available

Features that favour viral cause of sore throat (80–85% of cases)

- Children younger than 5 years of age (pre-school)

- Absence of the above features caused by bacterial infections including absence of petechiae on the palate and submandibular lymphadenopathy. Symptoms include rhinorrhoea, conjunctivitis, and cough occurring typically in a pre-school child who attends nursery. There is absence of dysphagia, abdominal pain, and headache

- Body temperature is either normal or between 38.0 °C and 39.0 °C

- Spontaneous resolution of symptoms is expected in about 48–72 h. No response to antibiotics

- Diagnosis is usually clinical. FBC: lymphocyte or lymphopenia, and leukopenia suggests viral aetiology. Rapid antigen test for GAS is negative. Viral study is not necessary

2. Other Causes of Pharyngo-Tonsillitis
   Peri-Tonsillar Abscess (Quinsy)

- Peri-tonsillar abscess is defined as a collection of pus located between the tonsillar capsule and the pharyngeal constrictor muscle.
- This is nowadays uncommon but it is the most common deep neck infection confined to one side.
- The abscess is a complication of tonsillitis that progresses to peri-tonsillitis and abscess.
- High fever (40–41 °C), toxic appearance, severe pain (odynophagia), difficulty in opening the mouth (trismus), drooling, uvula deviation, torticollis.
- The infection is usually caused by staphylococci. CT scan can confirm the diagnosis.

Scarlet Fever

- Scarlet fever results from certain strains of haemolytic streptococci producing an erythrogenic toxin. The rash is an erythematous punctiform eruption on the cheeks that blanches on pressure and spares the area around the mouth (peri-oral pallor). Initially the tongue has a thick white cover, which develops in a few days into typical strawberry tongue.
- There is essentially no difference between streptococcal tonsillitis and scarlet fever. Fever in both conditions usually ranges from 39 to 40.5 °C, peaking on the second day of illness. Without treatment, the temperature usually subsides on the fifth day, whereas penicillin therapy causes a rapid normalisation of temperature within 12–24 h.
- Diagnosis is confirmed by positive throat swab culture for streptococci, ASO titre rising 4-folds.

PFAPA (Periodic fever, aphthous stomatitis, pharyngitis, and adenitis)

- PFAPA is an auto-inflammatory condition due to abnormal innate immune system. It is the most common cause of periodic fevers that is characterised by high fever (39–40 °C) and rhythmic recurrences. PFAPA is mostly genetic, and generally remits in adolescence.

- Onset of symptoms of PFAPA usually occurs in early childhood (<5 years of age) with period fevers lasting 3–6 days and recurring every 3–4 weeks. The child is asymptomatic between the febrile episodes. Growth and development are normal.
- Diagnosis: clinical in individual who has a history of 3 or more episodes of fever that last up to 5 days and recur at regular intervals. CRP, WBC and pro-inflammatory cytokines are usually high during the febrile episodes.

Mononucleosis

- This Epstein–Barr (EB) virus infection predominately affects older children and adolescents, with a typical triad of abrupt onset of fever, pharyngo-tonsillitis, and cervical lymphadenopathy (Table 1.2). There are often petechiae at the junction of the hard and soft palate. Although pharyngo-tonsillitis of mononucleosis may resemble post-streptococcal infection, there is often a

TABLE 1.2 Clinical data and accuracy of laboratory data of infectious mononucleosis

Physical Features	%	Laboratory findings	%
Fever	100	EB-IgM	100
Lymphadenopathy	80	Monospot test	98
Pharyngitis	80	Liver enzymes transaminases ↑	90
Splenomegaly	50	>50% lymphocyte	50
Rash			
• Palatal petechiae	50		
• Exanthem	10		
Hepatomegaly	20		
Jaundice	5		
Airway obstruction	1–3.5		

characteristic grey membrane in mononucleosis instead of the typical multiple follicles of the later infection.

- Presentation may be as a pyrexia of unknown origin with fever as the only sign of the disease.
- A cytomegalovirus mononucleosis is characterised by prolonged fever, liver and haematological changes similar to those observed in Epstein–Barr infection. Heterophile antibodies are always absent. Pharyngitis is uncommon.
- Monospot test (sensitive in 90% and 95%); IgM for EBV is diagnostic.

Herpetic Gingivostomatitis

- This infection is caused by herpes simplex virus-1 that manifests with fever, malaise, and cervical lymphadenopathy. Children aged 6 months–6 years are mostly affected, peaking at 2–4 years.
- Typically the herpetic lesions consist of vesico-ulcerative eruption affecting the anterior part of the mouth: the gingiva, tongue, and cheek mucosa. The vesicles rapidly rupture and later covered by yellow–grey membranes.

Herpangina

- Herpangina is defined as the presence of ulcers on the anterior tonsillar pillars, soft palate, buccal mucosa, or uvula (In hand-foot-mouth disease the ulcers are on the tongue, buccal mucosa in addition to vesicular rashes on the palms and feet).
- Herpangina is caused by Coxsackievirus. The initial temperature is high up to 41 °C, associated with features include headache and vomiting.
- There are discrete punctuate vesicles, surrounded by erythematous rings on the soft palate, anterior pillars, and uvula.

TABLE 1.3 Diagnostic criteria of Kawasaki disease

Fever persisting for at least 5 days plus at least four of the following five:

1. Bilateral, painless conjunctival inflammation without exudates

2. Changes of the oropharynx mucosa, cracking lips, strawberry tongue

3. Acute unilateral non-purulent cervical lymphadenopathy >1.5 cm

4. Polymorphous rash, primarily truncal

5. Changes of extremities: oedema and/or erythema of hands and feet

Kawasaki Disease

- See diagnostic criteria in Table 1.3.
- Mucosal changes, including erythema, cracking, and peeling of the lips, strawberry tongue, and erythema of the oropharyngeal mucosa.
- Cervical lymphadenopathy with a minimum of one lymphnode of at least 1.5 cm in diameter, involvement being usually unilateral without suppuration.

3. Unilateral Tonsillitis

- Tonsillar asymmetry in appearance and size of normal tonsils is common in healthy children.
- Unilateral infection of the tonsils occurs as "peri-tonsillitis" or peri-tonsillar abscess (see above).
- Unilateral hyperplasia with the appearance of "tonsillitis", which does not resolve within a week following antibiotic therapy may suggest lymphoma.
- Another rare but important cause of unilateral tonsillitis is Plaut-Vincent angina caused by Treponema vincentii and fusiform bacteria. It affects mainly young adults but may affect children with poor oral hygiene and emotional stress. Clinical features include painful necrotising ulcerative membrane on oral mucosa and tonsils (pseudo-membrane) and halitosis.

4. Non-Infectious Pharyngo-Tonsillitis

- Neutropenia and Agranulocytosis

    - Neutropenia may present as absolute neutrophil count (ANC) of <1500 cells/μL, but is not significant unless the ANC decreases to <500 cells/μL. Agranulocytosis is a neutrophil count of <200 cells that can be caused by severe viral, bacterial or fungal infections.
    - Febrile neutropenia (defined as temperature of 38.3 °C or a temperature of 38.0 °C sustained over 1-h period) is detected in about two thirds of cases of neutropenia. Sore throat, gingivitis, and/or candida infection may be the first sign of the disease. Bacteraemia is detected in about a third of cases.

- Immunodeficiency Disorders

    - These are either primary (e.g. agamma-globulinaemia) or acquired (e.g. HIV, malnutrition, or chemotherapy) that manifest as sore throat due to candida (that can be an early and only manifestation) or herpes simplex infection. Other manifestations include gingivitis and parotid swelling.
    - Immunodeficiency disorders result from malfunction of the major components of the immune system (T-cells, B-cells, phagocytes, complements). There are commonly associated autoimmune disorders in about 25% of cases.

- Many systemic diseases (e.g., Crohn's disease) may present as extra-intestinal manifestations including ulcers in oral cavity, which may present as sore throat. It is essential to search for an underlying disease for any unexplained mouth ulcers, especially if severe, prolonged, multiple, or frequently recurring.

1.2 Stridor

Introduction/Core Messages
- Stridor is a harsh inspiratory sound caused by extra-thoracic airway obstruction, causing terrifying experience for the child and his parents. There is usually an associated upper respiratory tract infection (URTI). The onset of stridor is followed by barking cough, hoarseness, and varying degree of respiratory distress.
- Laryngo-tracheal obstruction causes inspiratory stridor, but severe obstruction produces inspiratory and expiratory stridor.
- The most important aspect of acute stridor is to differentiate between a life-threatening illness such as epiglottitis or foreign body and a relatively harmless croup caused by a viral infection.
- Croup is the most common diagnosis of stridor, which is based on easily recognisable clinical features. Despite this, alternative diagnoses should be considered. Diagnostic error may occur in differentiating various causes of acute and chronic stridor, particularly with atypical presentation.

Differential Diagnosis

Common	Rare
Laryngotracheobronchitis (croup)	Vascular ring
Spasmodic croup	Hypoglycaemia
Bacterial tracheitis	Epiglottitis
Laryngomalacia	Glottic stenosis
Haemangioma/laryngeal web	Hypocalcaemia
Foreign body	Intubation-associated stenosis
Angioneurotic oedema	

Misdiagnosis is due to:

1st mistake: failing to differentiate between the most common causes of acute stridor.

2nd mistake: failing to differentiate the causes of chronic stridor.

1. Causes of Acute Stridor

   Croup (laryngotracheobronchitis)

   Croup is a common cause of an upper respiratory tract obstruction of the subglottic area characterised by features shown in Table 1.4:

   Spasmodic croup

   This entity is of unknown aetiology, and is characterised by:

   - Onset is always at night.
   - Symptoms occur in a child who previously has been well without associated upper respiratory infection and

TABLE 1.4 Characteristic clinical features of croup

- The attack rate is highest in the second year of life (peak age: 6 months–3 years). Onset is sudden (usually at night) with loud inspiratory stridor, barking cough, hoarse voice, low-grade fever (occurring in 40% of cases), and a variable degree of respiratory distress, preceded by 24–72 h of a viral URTI. The infection commonly occurs in autumn and early winter

- Although symptoms often appear alarming, the infection is usually benign and self-limited, which persists for 2–6 days. Parainfluenza viruses account for about 75% of all isolates. Other pathogens include influenza A and B, adenovirus, and mycoplasma pneumonia

- It is unusual for the common croup to have hypoxia (pulse oximeter below 92%). If present, this would be an ominous sign requiring urgent attention. Inflammatory markers (WBC and CRP) are normal

- Symptoms improve with corticosteroids (dexamethasone or prednisolone) at 2 h with an effect lasting at least 24 h

who awakens at night with sudden, croupy cough and inspiratory stridor.
- Fever is absent.

Bacterial Tracheitis
This is an acute, potentially life-threatening bacterial infection. Characteristic features are:

- The infection is caused mostly by staphylococcal aureus of the tracheal mucosa. It begins as a viral-like illness or croup with stridor, but progresses rapidly with high fever, often producing thick purulent exudates, toxicity, and worsening respiratory distress.
- The diagnosis should be considered in any ill-looking child with adequate vaccination of Hib and who does not respond to nebulised adrenaline.

Epiglottitis
Epiglottitis is an acute bacterial infection characterised by:

- The infection has an abrupt onset with high fever (39–40.5 °C), respiratory distress, dysphagia, drooling, irritability, restlessness, anxiety, and a thick muffled voice. Patients appear very unwell, with higher degrees of fever and respiratory distress.
- The disease is caused by H. influenza type B, also known as Hib, that often manifests as septicaemia.
- Epiglottitis is rarely seen nowadays following Hib vaccines.
- There is usually leukocytosis and high CRP. BC yields the causing organisms.

Foreign Body

- In the absence of a viral respiratory tract infection, an acute stridor in an infant or toddler may suggest foreign body.
- Typical onset is a child 1–3 years of age with sudden choking and coughing that might be followed by symptoms-free period and thus be mistakenly as resolution.

- Chest X-ray is usually diagnostic.

Angioedema

- Angioedema (often with urticaria) is either allergic, idiopathic or hereditary causing often life-threatening airway obstruction depending on underlying cause and location. Clinical features include oedema of the face, tongue and lips, sore and itchy throat.
- Hereditary angioedema is characterised by recurrent episodes of swelling caused by mutation of the gene encoding CI inhibitors.
- Oedema is non-pitting, non-dependent and transient, which is either histamine-mediated or bradykinin-mediated. The latter is not mediated by IgE, and is not associated with urticaria.
- Prompt Adrenalin administration is life-saving.

2. Causes of Chronic Stridor
   Laryngomalacia

- Laryngomalacia is the most common cause of persistent stridor during infancy, typically appearing during the first few weeks of life. It is caused by soft tissue laxity of the larynx above the vocal cords, which collapses during inspiration. Stridor usually worsens during feeding, agitation, and supine position. The child has a normal cry (no hoarse voice indicating no vocal cord involvement) and normal cough.
- Condition is usually self-resolving. Parents can be reassured that recovery will occur aged 12–18 months, often even earlier.
- Laryngoscopy is required to confirm the inspiratory collapse of the larynx, and to exclude other causes of stridor.

Vascular Ring
- This is a congenital anomaly of the aorta resulting in complete or incomplete encirclement of the trachea, oesophagus or both. Incomplete vascular ring is often asymptomatic.

- The anomaly is rare representing approximately 1% of cardiovascular anomalies. Associated congenital heart diseases are common.
- Tracheal compression presents with respiratory symptoms (e.g., cough, wheezing, stridor) and/or gastrointestinal symptoms (e.g., dysphagia, feeding difficulty, vomiting).
- Diagnosis is by CT scan or MRI.

Tumours

- Other causes of chronic stridor include haemangioma, laryngeal web/cleft, adenoma, hamartoma, and papilloma, which cause symptoms during the first three months of life. Haemangioma is often associated with other haemangiomas on the head and neck.
- Symptoms are recurrent or persistent stridor, dyspnoea, hoarseness of the voice, and occasionally haemoptysis.
- Diagnosis by laryngoscopy and chest CT-scan.

Further Reading

Celmina M, Paule S. Stridor in children. Breathe. 2018;14(3):e111–7. https://doi.org/10.1183/20734735.017018.

El-Radhi AS. Clinical Manual of Fever in Children. 2nd edition, Chap 5, Springer Verlag; 2018.

Stelter K. Tonsillitis and sore throat in children. GMS Curr Top Otorhinolaryngol Head Neck Surg. 2014;13:Doc07.

Chapter 2
The Chest

2.1   Acute Shortness of Breath (Dyspnoea)

Introduction/Core Messages
- Dyspnoea is an "abnormal and uncomfortable awareness of one's own breathing. Common associated signs include cough, wheezing, tachypnoea and subcostal recession.
- Dyspnoea is a common symptom of a variety of cardio-pulmonary diseases. Asthma is the most common cause. Congestive cardiac failure is a rare but important cause of dyspnoea at any age of childhood.
- Children may describe dyspnoea as "getting easily tired", or "cannot keep up with other kids". It may occur spontaneously or during certain activities such as exercise or during feeding in infants.
- There is little knowledge as how to assess the severity of dyspnoea. Causes of dyspnoea are numerous and differentiating each cause from another is difficult. In addition, the differential diagnosis between cardiac and pulmonary causes of dyspnoea can be challenging. An incorrect diagnosis could result in the delayed detection of a serious illness and an unnecessary workout leading to wrong treatment.

© Springer Nature Switzerland AG 2021   15
A. S. El-Radhi, *Avoiding Misdiagnosis in Pediatric Practice*,
In Clinical Practice, https://doi.org/10.1007/978-3-030-41750-5_2

Differential Diagnosis
- Pulmonary
  - Asthma
  - Viral-induced wheeze/bronchiolitis
  - Pneumonia
  - Pulmonary oedema
  - Inhaled foreign body
- Cardiac
  - Congestive cardiac failure (CCF)
  - Myocarditis, pericarditis
  - Hypertrophic obstructive cardiomyopathy
- Metabolic acidosis such as diabetic ketoacidosis
- Neuromuscular diseases
- Psychogenic (mainly occurring in older children)

Misdiagnosis is due to:

1st mistake: failing to establish the presence and assessing the severity of dyspnoea.

2nd mistake: failing to establish diagnostic criteria of asthma as the most common cause of dyspnoea.

3rd mistake: failing to differentiate asthma from conditions mimicking asthma.

4th mistake: failing to recognise cardiac causes of dyspnoea.

5th mistake: failing to differentiate other less common causes of dyspnoea.

1. Assessing the Severity of Dyspnoea

   The assessment can be done by observation (e.g. facial appearance, speech flow), chest signs (e.g. respiratory rate, chest recession), and by tests to confirm the clinical impression (e.g. oxygen saturation, blood gases) (Table 2.1).

2. Establishing the Diagnosis of Asthma

   The diagnosis of asthma is established by adhering to the diagnostic criteria of asthma (Table 2.2) and by excluding conditions mimicking asthma (see next).

3. Conditions Mimicking Asthma

   Pneumonia
   - Pneumonia is defined as fever, clinical signs (cough, dyspnoea, tachypnoea, grunting and nasal flaring and

TABLE 2.1 The three degrees of severity of dyspnoea

Symptom	Mild	Moderate	Severe
Pulse rate	<120/min	120–170	>170
RR	<40/min	40–70	>70
SaO$_2$	>94%	90–94%	<90%
FEV1	>70%	50–70%	<50%
Drowsiness	No	No	Agitated or drowsy
Speech in	Sentences	Phrases	Difficult or unable to say a sentence
Subcostal	Mild	Moderate	Severe recession

SaO2 oxygen saturation, *FEV1* forced expiratory volume in 1 s of predicted for age

TABLE 2.2 Diagnostic criteria to establish the diagnosis of asthma

- Asthma is defined as a chronic inflammatory disorder of the airways characterised by bronchial hyper-responsiveness and variable airway obstruction. It is usually triggered by viral infection, exercise or inhaled allergens

- Clinically asthma is diagnosed by recurrent episodes of coughing, wheezing and chest tightness. These symptoms are commonly worse at night, particularly if asthma attacks are frequent and recurrent, and occurring in response to pet, cold and damp air exposure or emotion. Personal and family history of atopic diseases is common

- Spirometry and bronchodilator reversibility in a symptomatic child are useful investigation in the diagnostic workup. In doubtful diagnosis, quantification of eosinophilic count in sputum (<2% normal; >2%) is suggestive of eosinophilic inflammation. Total IgE, specific IgE and skin brick tests are often performed to support the diagnosis

referred pain) and chest x-ray infiltrates in a previously well child. Referred pain is when lower lobe pneumonia may cause lower abdominal pain mimicking acute appendicitis. Upper lobe pneumonia may cause meningism (increased CSF pressure, but CSF is otherwise normal).

- Findings include inspiratory crepitations and bronchial breathing on auscultation. Tachypnoea (>40/min aged >1 year, >50/min aged 2–12 months and >60/min aged <2 months) is the WHO defined criterion to diagnose pneumonia. A sign of pneumonia is grunting with flaring of alae nasi.
- Chest X-ray is diagnostic but it is often of limited value in distinguishing bacterial and viral. The presence of effusion and/or lobar consolidation suggests bacterial aetiology.
- Isolation of the pathogens causing pneumonia is usually not possible in practice. Bacterial culture from the pharyngeal area or expectorated sputum is unreliable. However, pathogens can be identified by: blood culture (positive in 10% of cases with bacterial pneumonia), high IgM, such as mycoplasma pneumoniae, respiratory secretion for rapid virus antigens (e.g. RSV, parainfluenza) and polymerase chain reaction (PCR) that has increasingly been used.

Cystic Fibrosis

- CF is the second most common chronic airway disease after asthma (incidence: 1 in 2500).
- CF is autosomal receive due to deficiency or dysfunction of the CF transmembrane conductance regulator anion channel.
- Clinical manifestations are characterised by multi-organ pathologies involving the respiratory (progressive lung disease), digestive (malabsorption, exocrine pancreatic insufficiency causing diabetes) and reproductive systems. There is little or no response to a short course of bronchodilator and steroids.

Primary Ciliary Dyskinesia (PCD)

- This ciliopathy is caused by genetic defects characterised by reduced muco-ciliary clearance of the airways. Clinical manifestations include early-onset persistent wet cough (bronchiectasis), persistent rhinitis, particularly neonatal rhinitis, chronic or recurrent otitis media (with or without hearing loss) and chronic sinusitis.

- Diagnosis of PCD can be confirmed by nasal nitric oxide measurement and electron microscopy. Siblings should also be tested.
- Situs inversus (Kartagener's syndrome) is present in about 50% of patients.

Primary Immunodeficiency

- Primary immunodeficiency disorders are hereditary disorders affecting either the innate or the adaptive immune system (e.g. combined immunodeficiency).
- Clinical manifestations include recurrent bacterial infections (e.g. otitis media, pneumonia, and gastroenteritis), more than one severe infection (e.g. meningitis, sepsis), oral mucocutaneous candidiasis, skin infections (e.g. abscess, pyoderma), and complication of vaccination (e.g. varicella, BCG). In addition, there is a high incidence of malignancies and autoimmune diseases.

Foreign Body (FB)

- FB occurs commonly in 1–3 year olds; the child being previously asymptomatic.
- There is usually sudden onset of respiratory distress with choking, cough, and asymmetric air entry or wheezing. Symptoms may persist or disappear for a period to present later with abscess formation, bronchiectasis or pneumonia. The symptom-free period may be mistaken as resolution.
- An obstructing object may occlude a bronchus (usually the right bronchus, which is straighter than left one), causing atelectasis that detected by dullness on lung percussion, diminished air entry on lung auscultation and typical opacity with well-defined margins on a chest x-ray.

Gastro-Oesophageal-Reflux

- Aspiration of gastric contents into respiratory tree causing symptoms such as vomiting causing recurrent aspiration that manifests as recurrent/persistent cough, wheezing, stridor, pneumonia.
- Inadequate weight gain, sleeping disturbance.
- Dystonic neck posturing (Sandifer syndrome).

4. Cardiac Dyspnoea

Heart diseases are either congenital = CHD (e.g. ventricular septal defect) or acquired (such as Kawasaki disease or myocarditis). CHD are detected by an antenatal ultrasonography, presence of a heart murmur, dyspnoea, cyanosis or heart failure.

Heart Failure (HF)

- Heart failure results from ventricular dysfunction, volume or pressure overload, either alone or in combination. Clinical features are shown in Table 2.3.
- The main causes of HF are congenital heart diseases and cardiomyopathy.
- A neonate who becomes dyspnoeic during feeding, a cardiac cause should be ruled out.
- An infant with no murmur detected at birth but found to have a murmur at the age of six weeks with respiratory distress is likely to have CCF due to large ventricular septal defect.

TABLE 2.3 Symptoms and signs of heart failure

Symptoms	Signs
Dyspnoea, fatigue	Persistent tachypnoea, tachycardia, 3rd or 4th heart sounds
	(Gallop), displaced apex, hepatomegaly, wheezing, basal
Chest pain	Lung crepitations, respiratory distress
Reduced exercise tolerance	Orthopnoea
Poor appetite	Poor growth

- The presence of a murmur, liver enlargement and relative tachycardia (in relation to the degree of dyspnoea) favours cardiac causes.
- An aid to differentiate cardiac from pulmonary dyspnoea is the hyperbaric oxygen test by breathing 100%.: In pulmonary diseases there will be a normalisation of the 02 saturation.

Cardiomyopathy

Cardiomyopathies are genetically heterogeneous disorders with many causes, primarily idiopathic and autosomal dominant inheritance. Dilated and hypertrophic cardiomyopathies occur most commonly in paediatric population.

Dilated Cardiomyopathy (DCM)

DCM is defined as decreased ventricular function secondary to subnormal myocardial systolic shortening. The wall thickness of the myocardium is normal. In additional to genetic causes, DCM may be idiopathic, caused by viral myocarditis (e.g. coxsackie, parvoviris B19 and Epstein-Barr viruses), inborn error of metabolism (e.g. carnithine deficiency), myopathies (e.g. Duchenne muscular dystrophy) and drugs (e.g. cyclophosphamide, anthracycline).

Clinical Presentation:

- Heart failure occurring in about 70–80% of cases. Infants and young children present with poor feeding, growth failure, exertional dyspnoea, fatigue, chest pain.
- Arrhythmia and sudden death.
- Diagnosis is established by history, including family history, ECG, chest x-ray, echocardiography and cardiac MRI. The degree of dilatation and ventricular dysfunction correlate with the risk of sudden death.

Hypertrophic Cardiomyopathy (HCM)

HCM may occur in infants of diabetic mothers, as secondary to obstructive CHD (e.g. severe aortic stenosis), or to storage diseases (e.g. glycogen storage disease) or idiopathic. The condition is mostly inherited as an autosomal dominant. Patients are either asymptomatic, mildly symptomatic or develop sudden cardiac arrest and die. It is known as a leading cause of sudden death in young athletes. Table 2.4 lists the main risk factors for sudden death. The cardiac hypertrophy is often massive and particularly involves the inter-ventricular septum.

Clinical findings include:

- Symptoms: Symptoms and signs of heart failure are rare with HCM. There may be no symptoms or occasionally exertional dyspnoea (exercise, physical activity), fatigue, chest pain or pressure, exertional syncope, and/or palpitation caused either by supraventricular tachycardia (SVT) or ventricular tachycardia (VT).
- Signs: displaced apex, gallop rhythm, prominent ventricular heave.
- There may be no murmur, or systolic ejection type of murmur of medium intensity (similar to the murmur of aortic stenosis). Murmur increases with standing or during the strain phase of Valsalva manoeuvre. Carotid pulsation is brisk and jerky.
- Once HCM has been diagnosed, immediate testing for HMC for all members of the family is required.
- Diagnosis as above with DCM.

TABLE 2.4 Risk factors for sudden death in patients with HCM	
	• Family history of HCM with sudden death of relatives
	• Recurrent episodes of syncope
	• Previous episodes of aborted cardiac arrest
	• A young age at first diagnosis (<30 years)
	• History of SVT or VT
	• Ventricular septal thickness >3 cm

5. Uncommon Causes of Dyspnoea
   - Metabolic diseases (e.g. congenital lactic acidosis, non-ketotic hyperglycaemia, organic acidaemia, lysosomal disorders and diabetic ketoacidosis) are often complicated by respiratory manifestations either at presentation or as late-onset features. Diagnosis is established by metabolic investigations.
   - Neuromuscular diseases (e.g. spinal muscular atrophy, muscular dystrophy and peripheral neuropathy) often lead to respiratory muscle weakness, insufficient ventilation and respiratory failure. Diagnosis is established by the history and muscle weakness.
   - Psychogenic dyspnoea may occur in healthy individual, usually older child or adolescent, or in a child with an underlying physical illness such as asthma, as a result of acute emotional stress. Associated features including giddiness, palpitation, tremor and hyperventilation. The latter symptom may result in washout of carbon dioxide thus inducing respiratory alkalosis and subsequently hypocalcaemia and carpopedal spasms of the fingers. Diagnosis is confirmed by ruling out physical illness.

2.2   Palpitation

Introduction/Core Messages
- Cardiologists may use the term of palpitation to describe an awareness of the heartbeat due to abnormality of the heart rhythm ranging from simple, benign ectopic atrial or ventricular beats to more important tachy-arrhythmias and life-threatening cardiac diseases. Patients may use the term to describe a perception or awareness of irregular, fast or skipped heartbeats or simple awareness of their pulse, particularly when it is fast or when lying on one side in bed. A young child who cannot explain the event by words may stop his or her normal activity, expressing discomfort or clinching the left side of the chest.

- Palpitation is usually a terrifying experience for children and for their parents. Evaluation must determine which patients only require reassurance and those who need investigation and treatment.
- Common causes of palpitation include tachycardia (such as supraventricular tachycardia, SVT), ectopic beats and cardiac diseases. Any palpitation with a history of syncope without warning is most likely of cardiac origin (ventricular tachycardia, VT). In such case, an urgent evaluation is essential.

Differential Diagnosis

Common	**Rare**
• Hyper-dynamic state (e.g. fever, exercise, anaemia)	Carcinoid syndrome
• Cardiac (e.g. premature atrial beats, SVT, arrhythmia)	Pheochromocytoma
• Anxiety	Thyrotoxicosis
• Drugs (e.g. bronchodilator, use of stimulants)	Hypoglycaemia

Misdiagnosis is due to:

1st mistake: failing to recognise benign non-cardiac causes of palpitation.

2nd mistake: failing to recognise benign cardiac causes of palpitation.

3rd mistake: failing to recognise serious cardiac causes of palpitation.

4th mistake: failing to recognise serious non-cardiac causes of palpitation.

1. Benign Non-cardiac Causes of Palpitation
   Hyper-dynamic state (or hyper-dynamic circulation)
   - Hyper-dynamic state is characterised by an increased heart rate and cardiac output above the normal limit at rest. This state occurs following exercise, fever and anaemia. The normal cardiac index in children is 3–5 l/min/m².
   - Drugs (e.g. caffeine, amphetamine) have to be considered in any older child with palpitation.

Anxiety
- Anxiety is frequently normal and adaptive emotional reaction in children to cope with challenging and stressful situation. Anxiety becomes pathological when it is excessive, difficult to control and interferes with social interaction, school performance or development. High level of anxiety is often associated with enlarged amygdala nuclei, which is considered as brain's emotion region.
- Palpitations are important diagnostic criteria for panic attacks and generalised anxiety disorders. Anxiety-related disorders include phobias and obsessive compulsive disorder (OCD).
- Phobias affect 1–2% of children. They are anxious usually under specific conditions as they try to avoid specific objects or situations that will automatically lead to anxiety. School phobia is an important type of phobia that usually a result of separation from the home and parents. Phobias usually become pathological if they interfere with social interaction and school performance.
- OCD is an anxiety disorder characterised by intrusive thoughts that produce apprehension, fear or worry leading to repetitive behaviours. Its incidence in adults is about 2%, and a third to a half of them report the onset of their disorder in childhood.

2. Benign Cardiac Causes of Palpitation
   Arrhythmias can be harmless or life-threatening events such as those originating below the bundle of His. Arrhythmias that cause palpitation are usually tacharrhythmias as shown in the Fig. 2.1.
   Sinus Tachycardia. This is the most common arrhythmia in children occurring after fever, exercise, anaemia, hypovolaemia and medications such as stimulants. It is distinguished from SVT by:

   - Tachycardia of 100–140 beats per min (bpm) in older children and 160–180 bpm in infants.
   - The presence of sinus P wave preceding every QRS complex in the ECG.

Tachycardia

Supra-ventricular	Ventricular
↙	↘
Sinus tachycardia	Premature ventricular complexes
Supra-ventricular tachycardia	Ventricular tachycardia
Ectopic beats (extra-systole)	Ventricular fibrillation
Atrial flutter	

FIG. 2.1 Simplified classification of the main tachycardia

Paroxysmal Supraventricular Tachycardia (SVT) is a regular rhythm at a rate of 180–300 beats/min. SVT is caused by impulses from the atrioventricular (AV) node re-entering the atria. It is characterised in children by:

- Tachycardia >220 bpm under 1 year of age and >180 bpm > 1 year of age narrow QRS with absent P.
- ECG is characterised by regular narrow QRS with absent P waves. About 25% of children with SVT have Wolff Parkinson-White syndrome (a delta wave, short PR-interval, wide QRS complex).
- Infants often present with signs of cardiac failure, in addition to irritability, crying, fatigue, poor appetite. Older child presents with dizziness, dyspnea in addition to palpitation.

Ectopic beats (Extra-systole) are common everyday findings clinically and in ECG records:

- They are usually atrial in nature and rarely ventricular in nature.
- Isolated ectopic beats are of no clinical significance, but multiple frequent beats are occasionally associated with organic heart disease.

Atrial Flutter may occur in neonates and is usually not associated with heart disease. Atrial flutter in older children is often associated with CHD such as mitral insufficiency that causes atrial enlargement. It may also be associated with chromosomal anomaly and hydrops fetalis. Characteristic features are:

- Atrial beats 250–400 bpm; the ventricles respond to every 2nd–4th atrial beat.
- ECG usually shows normal P waves and QRS complexes, rapid and regular atrial flutter waves.
- Severe and prolonged atrial flutter can cause heart failure.
- Defibrillation converts the flutter to sinus rhythm immediately.

Premature Ventricular Complexes (PVCs) (extra-systole) may be caused by febrile illness, anxiety or ingestion of drugs such as stimulants. They are characterised by:

- Premature, wide QRS complexes that are not preceded by a P wave, often followed by compensatory pause.
- When frequent they assume a definite rhythm, e.g. alternating with normal rhythm (bigeminy) or occurring after two normal beats (trigeminy).
- Benign PVCs should be distinguished from more serious complexes by their disappearance during the tachycardia of exercise. Those PVCs which do not disappear are categorised as serious and need further investigation.

3. Serious Cardiac Causes of Palpitation
   Ventricular Tachycardia is uncommon, life-threatening event in children and characterised by:

- Likely to occur in children with underlying cardiac lesion such as cardiomyopathy or following cardiac surgery.
- Regular rhythm of >120 bpm with a wide QRS complex (>0.08s) without P waves.

Long QT syndrome is either autosomal dominant inherited (Romano–Ward syndrome), autosomal recessive (Jervell-Lange-Nielson syndrome) or acquired (myocarditis or electrolyte disturbance).

- It is found in approximately 1 in 2000 birth and causes 10% of SIDS.

- Is an important cause of loss of consciousness (syncope) and may mimic epilepsy and sudden cardiac death. Child may recover immediately after the episode or die during the event.
- A heart rate-corrected QT-interval > 470 milliseconds supports the diagnosis, whereas a QT-interval >440 ms is suspicious.

Dilated Cardiomyopathy (DCM): (See Cardiac Dyspnoea: 2.1 Acute Shortness of Breath)
Hypertrophic Cardiomyopathy (HCM) (See Cardiac Dyspnoea: 2.1 Acute Shortness of Breath)

4. Serious Non-cardiac Causes of Palpitation
Pheochromocytoma

- Pheochromocytoma is rare but potentially fatal unless recognised and treated. Classical presentation is episodic sweating, headache, chest pain and palpitation. Hypertension is an important finding.
- Tumour is mainly located in the adrenal medulla (up to 95%), and uncommonly in the paravertebral area.
- Diagnosis is established by finding increased urinary catecholamines and imaging of the adrenal glands.

Carcinoid Syndrome (CS)

- CS is a paraneoplastic syndrome frequently associated with neuro-endocrine tumours.
- Classical presentation includes episodic flushing, associated with hypotension, tachycardia, diarrhoea, dyspnea due to bronchospasm and cardiac manifestation (Tricuspid, mitral or pulmonary regurgitation).
- Diagnosis is confirmed by increased urinary 24 h of 5-HIAA.

Hyperthyroidism
Presentation is highly variable but usually includes:

- Motor activity, emotional lability, irritability and easily crying, loss of concentration and weight loss.
- Findings include tremor, goitre, exophthalmos with lagging of the upper eyelid as the eyes look downward.

2.3   Chest Pain

Introduction/Core Messages
- Chest pain is the second most frequent cause of referral to the paediatric cardiologists after cardiac murmur. The vast majority of causes of chest pain are non-cardiac.
- Idiopathic chest pain is the most common cause of chest pain, occurring in 20–45% of cases. Condition is defined by absence of cause after thorough history, physical examination and laboratory testing.
- Chronic (lasting >6 months) or recurrent episodes of chest pain without abnormal findings is likely to be psychogenic. This cause accounts for 5–10% of cases.
- Serious attention has to be given to children who present with abnormal physical examination findings, abnormal ECG, exertional chest pain (after excluding respiratory disease), associated palpitation or family history of cardiomyopathy. Referral for further evaluation is essential.

Differential Diagnosis

CommonNon-cardiac causes	RareCardiac causes
Idiopathic	Severe aortic stenosis
Anxiety or stress	Pericarditis
Costochondritis	Hypertrophic cardiomyopathy
Direct trauma to the chest	Long QT syndrome
Pulmonary (pneumonia, asthma, pleurisy)	Paroxysmal supraventricular tachycardia
Acid reflux	Aortic aneurysm (e.g. Marfan's syndrome)
Acute chest pain (e.g. Sickle cell anaemia)	

Misdiagnosis is due to:

1st mistake: failing to recognise common non-cardiac causes of chest pain.

2nd mistake: failing to differentiate non-cardiac causes of chest pain from those of cardiac origin.

1. Non-Cardiac Causes of Chest Pain
   - The vast majority of cases with chest pain are idiopathic, musculoskeletal, respiratory, or gastrointestinal or psychogenic (Table 2.5).
   - Typical for non-cardiac cause of chest pain: sharp quality, of short duration and unrelated to exercise.
   - Costochondritis (Tietze's syndrome), frequently caused by viral infection, is characterised by localised swelling of the costo-chondral, costo-sternal or sterno-clavicular joints, mostly involving the 2nd and 3rd ribs. Chest movements or taking a deep breath may worsen the pain. Condition is more common in girls.

2. Cardiac Causes of Chest Pain
   - Warning symptoms and signs that may signal cardiac aetiology for chest pain are shown in Table 2.6.
   - Cardiac causes of chest pain are rare (around 1–2% of cases) which include pericarditis, myocarditis, SVT, hypertrophic and dilated cardiomyopathy (Table 2.7).
   - Chest pain in infancy is difficult to diagnose. An infant who presents with sweating, restlessness and crying (as equivalent signs for expressing chest pain) may have a serious cardiac disease, e.g. acute chest syndrome in SCA, or anomalous origin of the coronary arteries.
   - Chest pain of cardiac origin manifests as a deep heavy pressure, choking or squeezing sensation, and it is usually triggered by exercise. It is not sharp and is not affected by respiration.

TABLE 2.5 Non-cardiac causes of chest pain

Causes	Diagnostic consideration
Idiopathic	Chest pain typically short for few min Normal physical examination, chest x-ray, ECG, echocardiography, and 24-Holter monitoring
Musculoskeletal	Chest muscle tenderness, difficulty in breathing
Respiratory	Associated wheezing dyspnoea, tachypnoea
GO-reflux*	Vomiting, chest pain in relation to food intake. Diagnosis by ambulatory 24-h oesophageal pH testing
Acute chest syndrome	Features resemble pneumonia: fever, x-ray infiltration
Psychogenic	Older children affected, history of recurrent dyspnoea, hyperventilation and panic episodes

* *Go-reflux* Gastro-oesophageal reflux

TABLE 2.6 Warning features that need further cardiac evaluation

History	Physical examination	ECG findings
Palpitation, chest pain, syncope	Tachycardia/ tachypnoea	Atrial or ventricular hypertrophy
Known cardiac arrhythmia, dyspnoea/syncope	Pathological murmur, gallop rhythm	Long QTc interval >440 ms
Positive family history in 1st Irregular rhythm, or 2nd degree relative of cardiomyopathy		

TABLE 2.7 Common cardiac causes of chest pain

Pericarditis/myocarditis	History of viral infection at the onset of cardiac disease (e.g. Coxsakie). Fever, dyspnoea, chest pain, arrhythmia, fatigability ECG changes, leukocytosis, high CRP. Viral diagnosis by PCR from blood
Rheumatic myocarditis/ pericarditis	Clinical features as above. In addition to rheumatologic features
Cardiomyopathies	Dyspnoea, chest pain, fatigability, signs of cardiomegaly, e.g. displaced apex and heart failure
Arrhythmia	(See the above section of Palpitation)

- When the presentation of chest pain/discomfort is associated with syncope, cardiac cause needs to be considered such as aortic stenosis, atrial myxoma (associated with tuberous sclerosis), hypertrophic cardiomyopathy, long QT syndrome and SVT with very rapid heart rate.
- Patients with Marfanoid appearance and chest pain require close attention because they are at risk of dilatation of the ascending aorta and dissecting aneurysm.

2.4   Heart Murmur

Introduction/Core Messages

- Examination of a child's heart includes palpation of pulses, for thrill, and apex (for evidence of displacement as a sign of heart enlargement). The brachial pulse should be palpated, not the radial one (The closer to the heart the pulse the better is its quality). The majority of patients with coarctation have weak or absent femoral and dorsalis pedis pulses.
- Heart murmur is a very common finding and is detected in over 50% of school children. It is usually physiological benign. Peak age of its detection 3–6 years of age.
- Electronic stethoscope coupled with phono-spectrographic analysis improve the accuracy of heart murmur evaluation.
- Although the vast majority of heart murmur are benign, parents often believe that a heart murmur is a sign of structural heart abnormality. They believe their child would be at increased risk of heart disease later in life.
- The distinction between innocent and pathological murmurs is often not easy in medical practice. The clinical significance of misinterpreting a physiological murmur can lead to unnecessary, complicated and time-consuming diagnostic procedures. This is why the recognition of innocent murmurs is essential. On the other hand, missing a pathological murmur may be lethal. This section provides detailed information to enable clinicians to differentiate innocent from pathological murmurs.

Differential Diagnosis of Types of Murmur

Common	Rare
Innocent (functional) murmur	Diastolic murmur
Systolic ejection murmur	Continuous murmur
Pansystolic murmur	
Venous hum	

Misdiagnosis is due to:

1st mistake: failing to accurately diagnose innocent murmur.

2nd mistake: failing to establish the diagnosis of a pathological murmur.

3rd mistake: confusion venous hum with a continuous murmur.

1. Recognition of innocent murmur

   Recognising innocent murmur is important to reduce unnecessary referral and misdiagnosis. Clinical criteria of an innocent murmur are shown in Table 2.8.

2. Recognition of pathological murmur

   The disappearance of a heart murmur on standing is a reliable clinical tool to rule out pathological murmurs in children. Characteristic features of pathological murmurs are shown in Tables 2.10 and 2.11.

3. Venous hum

   The greatest significance of venous hum is the mistaking of a normal phenomenon such as venous hum for a pathological murmur such as patent ductus arteriosus (PDA). Diagnostic criteria are shown in Table 2.12.

TABLE 2.8 Criteria for diagnosing innocent murmurs

- Short systolic ejection, low intensity, not pansystolic murmur, diastolic murmur or greater in intensity than grade II (Table 2.9)

- No or insignificant radiation to the apex, base or back

- It changes intensity being louder in supine position and disappearance in standing

- Murmur quality is vibratory or musical

- Low to middle left sternal border location (3rd to 4th intercostal space)

- It is grade 1 or II in intensity that increases with tachycardia

- Absence of symptoms and signs of heart disease

TABLE 2.9 Intensity grades of a murmur

• Grade 1	Difficult to hear, softer than the heart sounds
• Grade 2	Intensity equal to heart sounds
• Grade 3	Louder than the heart sounds, no thrill
• Grade 4	Loud murmur associated with thrill
• Grade 5	Is heard with only the edge of the stethoscope

TABLE 2.10 Clinical features that suggest pathological murmur

- Diastolic or late systolic murmur

- Loud murmur > 2/6 in intensity

- Continuous murmur with the exception of venous hum

- A murmur that sounds like a breath sound

- A murmur at the pulmonary area with fixed splitting of the second sound

- Associated with any symptom or sign of heart disease such as fatigue, shortness of breath, tachypnoea, hepatomegaly

TABLE 2.11 Diagnostic features of each pathological murmur

Murmur	Differentiating it from innocent murmur/ venous hum
Pansystolic (VSD, MI, AI)	Murmur is pansystolic, loud, presence of thrill, strong radiation
Ejection type, left (ASD, PS)	Fixed 2nd sound, murmur is louder and of longer duration than IM, radiates to axilla and back, ejection click is present
Ejection type, right (AS, CA)	Loud and harsh murmur, radiates to jugular vein and carotids, ejection click is present
Diastolic (AR, PI)	High frequency, blowing, starting after the S2 and end before S1; more difficult to hear and diagnose
Continuous (PDA)	Murmur is heard nearly all over the thorax, no change of its loudness with change of body position

VSD ventricular septal defect, *MI* mitral insufficiency, *AI* aortic incompetence, *ASD* atrial septal defect, *PS* pulmonary stenosis, *AS* aortic stenosis, *CA* coarctation of aorta, *AR* aortic regurgitation, *PI* pulmonary incompetence, *PDA* patent ductus arteriosus

TABLE 2.12 Characteristic features of venous hum

- Venous hum is a continuous murmur that commonly appears aged 3–8 years, and is caused by vibration of the internal jugular vein walls

- It is best heard at the base of the neck just below the right clavicle

- It is mostly prominent in sitting position and when turning the head to the opposite direction

- Venous hum is best heard just below the clavicle. It disappears when the child:

  – lies supine, or

  – turns his/her head to the other side, or

  – The jugular vein being compressed on the affected side

Further Reading

Bejic E, Bejic Z. Accidental heart murmur. Med Arch. 2017;71(4):284–7.

Friedman KG, Alexander ME. Chest pain and syncope in children: a practice approach to the diagnosis of cardiac disease. J Pediatr. 2013;163(3):896–901.

Gaaloul I, Riabi S, Harrath R, et al. Coxsackievirus B detection in cases of myocarditis, myo-pericarditis, pericarditis and dilated cardiomyopathy in hospital patients. Mol Med Rep. 2014;10(6):2011–8.

Lefort B, Cheyssac E, Soule N, et al. Auscultation while standing: a basic and reliable method to rule out a pathologic heart murmur in children. Ann Fam Med. 2017;15(6):523–8.

Chapter 3
The Ear

3.1 Deafness/Impaired Hearing

Introduction/Core Messages

- Hearing impairment is either conductive or sensorineural.
- The conductive hearing impairment is very common: At least half of the preschool children have one or more episodes of otitis media with effusion (OME), causing varying degree of hearing impairment, usually mild (26–40 dB).
- The incidence of congenital sensorineural is approximately 1–2:1000 neonates, usually severe (61–80 dB) or profound (>80 dB). Cytomegalovirus (CMV) is the leading non-genetic cause of this type of hearing loss.
- Risk factors for hearing impairment include genetic hearing loss, low gestation <32 weeks, pre-auricular pits or tags, branchial cysts, heterochromia of the iris, prolonged jaundice, ototoxic drugs, hypoxic ischaemic encephalopathy, congenital infections (CMV, rubella, syphilis), and neonatal meningitis.
- The detection of hearing loss in children is of paramount importance to avoid speech-language delay,

© Springer Nature Switzerland AG 2021
A. S. El-Radhi, *Avoiding Misdiagnosis in Pediatric Practice*,
In Clinical Practice, https://doi.org/10.1007/978-3-030-41750-5_3

communication problems, social and emotional isolation, and behavioural difficulties. This section provides information how to detect hearing loss and lists conditions associated with it.

Differential Diagnosis

Common	Rare
Neonatal deafness	Acoustic neuroma
congenital sensorineural hearing loss	Alport syndrome
Prematurity (weight <1800 g)	Osteopetrosis
Hypoxic-ischaemic injury	Osteogenesis imperfecta
Infection (meningitis, CMV)	Congenital syphilis
Hyperbilirubinaemia	
Ototoxic drugs (e.g., aminoglycoside)	
Intensive care unit graduates	
Syndromes (e.g., Pendred, Waardenburg)	
Acquired	
Otitis media with effusion (OME) = glue ears	
Trauma	
Infection	

Misdiagnosis is due to:

1st mistake: failing to diagnose congenital deafness.

2nd mistake: failing to identify common underlying causes of congenital deafness.

3rd mistake: failing to establish diagnostic criteria for otitis media with effusion (OME).

4th mistake: little knowledge on other acquired causes of deafness.

1. Diagnosing Congenital Deafness

- It is estimated that 1–2 newborns/1000 live births have varying degrees of bilateral sensorineural hearing loss, usually either severe (61–80 dB) or profound (>80 dB) (Table 3.1). The incidence of hearing loss in older children and adolescents is about 3.5%.
- Causes include genetic-hereditary (about 70%), syndromes, congenital infection (CMV, rubella), craniofacial anomalies, and malformation of the inner ears.
- Risk factors predisposing to hearing loss include positive family history, prematurity, admission to an intensive care unit, assisted ventilation, and medication use (ototoxic drugs such as aminoglycosides, diuretics). These children require regular follow-ups. Hearing test should be performed prior to hospital discharge.
- Since March 2006, all babies born in England are offered hearing screening with otoacoustic emissions = OAE. In case of no response to OAE, automated brain stem response = ABR enables early detection and early intervention to prevent delays in speech and language development. ABR is the most reliable screening device. Pure tone audiometry is suitable between 6 and 24 months.
- Congenital or genetically determined hearing loss may escape neonatal screening testing and deteriorate during the first 2 years of life.

2. Diagnosing Underlying Causes of Congenital Deafness
   Once a diagnosis of congenital hearing loss is made, the search for aetiological diagnosis is required.

TABLE 3.1 Degrees of hearing loss

• <25 dB	Normal hearing
• 26–40 dB	Mild hearing loss
• 41–60 dB	Moderate hearing loss
• 61–80 dB	Severe hearing loss
• >81 dB	Profound hearing loss

Genetic Hearing Loss

- The majority of hearing loss has a genetic basis, most often due to a single gene defect that can affect any component of the hearing pathway. Around 70% have genetic basis without a syndrome, i.e. without dysmorphic features including normal appearance of the external ears. First line genetic testing includes screening for mutations in GJB2 and GJB6 genes.
- A positive family history of hearing loss suggests a genetic involvement. Example are: Pendred syndrome (associated with hypothyroidism and goiter), Alport syndrome (glomerular renal disease with eye defect), Usher syndrome (associated with retinitis pigmentosa), and Waardenburg syndrome (associated with depigmentation of the skin and hair). Autosomal recessive hearing loss without a syndrome accounts for the majority of cases followed by autosomal dominant inheritance.

Craniofacial Anomalies

- Anomalies include pre-auricular pits and tags, branchial cysts or fistula, cleft palate, mandibular hypoplasia, and macroglossia. These can cause an upper airway obstruction and later sleep disorder.
- Imaging of the ears is required in all cases of craniofacial anomalies.

Cytomegalovirus (CMV) Infection

- This infection is the most common non-genetic cause of sensorineural congenital infection occurring as a perinatal infection via trans-placental route. It affects about 1% of neonates in the USA. Any child with congenital sensorineural deafness should be tested for CMV infection.
- Children with congenital CMV infection are usually born asymptomatic (about 90%), and about 10% are symptomatic with intra-uterine growth retardation, cerebral palsy, seizures, periventricular calcification and cerebral ventriculomegaly. Other manifestations include haematological (thrombocytopenia), ocular (microphthalmia, cataract, retinal, blindness) and hepatic (jaundice, hepatosplenomegaly) abnormalities.

- Virological identification of CMV should be established in the first 3 weeks of life in order to consider the infection as congenital. The virus can be identified from saliva, urine, and PCR-based blood spots.

Congenital Rubella (Rubella Syndrome)

- This infection is prevalent in countries without rubella vaccination program. Infection usually occurs before 3 months of age.
- Rubella infection causes hearing loss, as is the most common complication, congenital heart disease, cataract, microcephaly, jaundice, hepatosplenomegaly, thrombocytopenia, and leukopenia.
- Diagnosis is made by IgM and rising IgG titer, PCR in blood and urine during the first 2–3 weeks of life.

Other Infections

- These infections include herpes simplex (causing skin vesicles, microcephaly, cranial calcification), toxoplasmosis (causing visual, e.g., interstitial keratitis, motor and cognitive abnormalities), and syphilis infections (causing anaemia, splenomegaly, snuffles, and bone lesions such as osteochondritis, periostitis).
- Herpes infection is diagnosed by PCR or immunofluorescence testing from lesion scrapings, or electron microscopy; toxoplasmosis is diagnosed by IgM or PCR testing; and syphilis is diagnosed by IgM, PCR or venereal disease research laboratory (VDRL).

3. Diagnostic Criteria of Otitis Media with Effusion (OME)

- OME is as an inflammation of the middle ear with collection of non-purulent fluid behind an intact tympanic membrane (TM).
- OME is common. Following suppurative otitis media, effusion will be present in:
  - 80% of cases at 2 weeks
  - 40% at 1 month
  - 20% at 2 months
  - 10% at 3 months

TABLE 3.2 Typical presentation of a child with OME

Risk factors	Age 2–5 years attending a day-care nursery
	Exposure to tobacco smoke
	Adenoid hypertrophy
	Down syndrome, cleft palate
Presentation	History of otitis media
	Hearing impairment and/or speech delay
	Poor school performance (lack of concentration)
	Behavioural and sleep problems
Findings (pneumatic otoscopy)	TM: reduced movement, opaque, yellow or blue colour due to accumulation of fluid in the middle ear, turning to a brown colour when OME becomes chronic
Hearing loss	Usually mild: 15–30 dB
Diagnostic tool	Audiometry, tympanometry (showing flat curve)

TM tympanic membrane

- The diagnosis of OME is made by the history, examination, and supportive investigation (Table 3.2).
- Although the insertion of grommets for OME is effective in improving language acquisition, this effect lasts as long as the grommets are patent. Long-term benefits are not certain.

4. Other Acquired Causes of Hearing Impairment
   Infection

- Infections causing hearing loss include viral and bacterial meningitis, HIV, toxoplasmosis, and acquired infection CMV (see above).

   Acoustic Neuroma

- A child with unilateral progressive deafness, vertigo, and tinnitus should be suspected as having acoustic neuroma with ipsilateral location to the affected ear.

- Children with neurofibromatosis are at higher risk of developing this tumour.

Ototoxic Drugs

- Ototoxic drugs include Aminoglycosides (e.g., gentamicin), diuretics (Furosemide), and chemotherapeutical agents (e.g., Cisplatin).
- Ototoxic drugs tend to cause more damage to the vestibular branch of the 8th cranial nerve (tinnitus and imbalance) than the auditory one. Therefore hearing loss is usually minimal.

Autoimmune-Associated Hearing Loss

- This disorder is defined as a condition of a bilateral, asymmetric, sensorineural hearing loss caused by "uncontrolled" immune response.
- There is often a vestibular involvement and patients present with loss of balance and tinnitus.

3.2 Earache (Otalgia)

Introduction/Core Messages
- The ear receives its sensory innervation from 4 cranial nerves (V, Vll, lX, X) and two cervical nerves (C2 and C3).
- The pain usually arises from inflammation in the middle or external canal of the ear. In infancy, the pain usually manifests as irritability and tenderness when the ear is rubbed or touched.
- Otalgia is one of the most common reasons for seeking medical attention. Although otalgia is usually associated with pain from inside the ear (otogenic otalgia), pain may also originate from outside the ear (referred otalgia).
- In contrast to adults, referred pain from outside the ears is common in paediatrics, occurring via five main sources: via trigeminal nerve (sensory distribution of

the face); via facial nerve (teeth, most commonly the upper molars or temporomandibular joint); via glossopharyngeal nerve (tonsillitis, pharyngitis); via vagus nerve (laryngopharynx or oesophagus), or via 2nd to 3rd cervical vertebrae. In these cases patients have a normal otological examination.

- Although pain originating from the ear is a straight-forward diagnosis, recognition of pain from outside the ears is often ignored or undiagnosed. In addition to the causes of referred otalgia, the section provides clear diagnostic tools to differentiate bacterial from viral causes of this common complaint.

Differential Diagnosis

Common	Rare
Infective otitis media	Mastoiditis
Infective otitis externa	Trigeminal neuralgia
Referred pain (tooth ache, pharyngitis)	Temporomandibular arthritis
Foreign body	Ramsey Hunt syndrome (herpes zoster oticus)
Infected eczematous dermatitis	Perichondritis/chondritis
Barotitis media (e.g., Flying)	Osteoma
Impacted cerumen	Bullous myringitis

Misdiagnosis occurs because of:

1st mistake: failing to differentiate otogenic otalgia from referred otalgia.

2nd mistake: failing to distinguish bacterial from viral OM

3rd mistake: failing to differentiate the main causes of otogenic otalgia.

1. Otogenic Versus Referred Otalgia

   • Otoscopic examination usually detects the reason for the otalgia. Otogenic otalgia manifests as either otitis media (OM) or external otitis (EO). In case of otalgia due to OM, the tympanic membranes (TM) are hyperaemic with varying degree of bulging and possibly otorrhoea. There are commonly systemic manifestations such as fever, anorexia and malaise. Typically there is no associated middle ear effusion. In case of otitis externa (OE), the otalgia tends to be more severe than that of OM. The ear canal is usually red and oedematous; pustule or furuncle is often a common finding. The ear canal in swimmer's ear is diffusely red (see also otitis externa below).

   • Diagnosis of referred otalgia rests on absence of the above ear findings. It is important to note that any pathology affecting the sensory pathways of 4 cranial nerves (V, VII, IX and X) and two upper cervical nerves (C2 and C3) can causes referred otalgia. For example, trigeminal otalgia of the 5th cranial nerve is known to cause referred otalgia.

2. Differentiating Bacterial from Viral OM

   • Acute OM is one of the most common infectious diseases in childhood with a peak incidence 6–24 months, by which age around 90% of children had at least one episode of OM. Distinction between bacterial and viral OM should be made (Table 3.3). Only 4% of children persist with fever lasting longer than 48 h. Persistent fever suggests a viral cause, resistant bacteria, unsuitable antibiotic, or a complication of OM.

3. Other Causes of Otogenic Otalgia
   Otitis Externa (OE)

   • In contrast to the microbial aetiology of otitis media, OE is often caused by swimming or diving. Moisture, humidity, and water in the ear remove the protective layer of cerumen leading to infection with various bacteria.

TABLE 3.3 Differentiating bacterial from viral OM

Category	In favour of bacterial OM	In favour of viral OM
Age	6–4 months (especially <6 months)	>24 months
Pain	AOM with moderate to severe otalgia	Mild otalgia
Fever	Sudden and high >39.0 °C	<39.0 °C
URTI	Preceding URTI	Presence of an URTI
TM	Mild-moderate bulging/ severe hyperaemia	No bulge or severe hyperaemia
Discharge	Purulent discharge	No or non-purulent discharge
Risk factors	e.g. immunodeficiency, if present	No risk factors
Antibiotics	Good response	Poor response
Complication	e.g. mastoiditis	No complication

OM otitis media; *TM* tympanic membrane; *URTI* upper respiratory tract infection

- While perichondritis indicates infection of the surrounding tissue of the auricular cartilage (the outer third of the ear canal), chondritis indicates infection of the cartilage itself. This is usually caused by trauma, such as ear piercing.
- Ramsay-Hunt syndrome occurs by reactivation of the herpes zoster virus (HZV) at the geniculate ganglion. The virus can infect the external auditory canal, eardrum and the inner ear often leading (in about 50%) to permanent hearing loss. Clinically the syndrome presents with severe ear pain, vesicles on the pinna and in the external ear canal and features of peripheral facial palsy. In immunocompromised individuals the infection is severe and could be fatal.

- Furunculosis, caused by staphylococcal infection of the hair follicle, can affect only the cartilaginous outer hair-containing the outer one-third of the ear. The pain is severe in association with local tenderness. Movement of jaw and pinna is painful.
- Fungal infection (Aspergillus or candida) of the external canal causes ear discomfort and intense itching.
- Some topical otic preparations (neomycin, colistin, polymyxin), that used to treat OE, can cause contact dermatitis which manifests as erythema, vesiculation, and oedema.

Barotitis

- Barotitis occurs through damage to the middle ear due to ambient pressure changes. This may occur during a sudden ambient pressure increase subsequent to descent of an airplane or deep-sea diving in the presence of dysfunctional tube.
- Parents should be advised to be cautious to fly if their child has an URTI or allergy as the relative negative pressure in the middle ear may result in retraction of the eardrums causing pain and possibly bleeding in the middle ear.

Foreign Body, Impacted Cerumen

- Small children are commonly fond of inserting any small items into the ears such as papers, stones, or seeds. Accidently, an insect enters the ear canal without being noticed.
- Cerumen, secreted by glands in the external canal, has a useful lubricating role of the external canal as well as entrapping foreign bodies. When accumulated, it forms a solid brown or yellowish mass occluding the ear canal.
- Both foreign body and impacted cerumen cause impairment of hearing, blockage feeling, and sometimes tinnitus, and disturbance of balance due to pressure on the tympanic membrane.

Cholesteatoma: See under Ear Discharge

3.3   Ear Discharge (Otorrhoea)

Introduction/Core Messages
- Ear discharge (Otorrhoea) is an unpleasant experience for a child. It can cause bad malodour and has a negative impact on children's quality of life and school performance.
- Children are at high risk for otitis media and ear discharge if they are in a smoking environment, attending a day care, having frequent colds, allergic rhinitis or adenoid hypertrophy. In neonates, risk factors of OM include nasotracheal intubation for more than 7 days, cleft palate and prematurity.
- After an acute OM, about 40% of children develop otitis media effusion (OME) that persist for a month; and 10% have a persistent OME after three months.
- The most serious complication of OM is intracranial suppurative infections including meningitis, subdural empyema, and otogenic brain abscess. For this reason clinicians should be aware of all causes of ear discharge.

Differential Diagnosis

Common	Rare
Suppurative otitis media	Cholesteatoma
Infective otitis externa	Infected foreign body
Seborrhoeic dermatitis	CSF otorrhoea
Otorrhoea from tympanostomy tube	Herpes zoster
Chronic suppurative OM	Mastoiditis
	Tumour (e.g., rhabdomyosarcoma, eosinophilic granuloma)

Misdiagnosis is due to:

1st mistake: failing to distinguish common from rare causes of ear discharge.

2nd mistake: failing to establish the underlying sources of these discharges.

1. Causes of Ear Discharge

Common Causes

- Most ear discharges originate from either bacterial OM or OE, and therefore the discharge is usually purulent yielding positive bacterial culture such as S pneumonia, H influenzae, or Moraxella catarrhalis. History of symptoms is short and includes previous URTI, otalgia, and fever.
- A persistent ear discharge beyond two weeks is mostly caused by chronic suppurative OM. Culture is likely to yield Pseudomonas, Staphylococci, or Proteus. Otorrhoea is commonly associated with hearing loss and perforated tympanic membrane.
- Insertion of grommets is often associated with ear discharge (see below).

Uncommon Causes

- Any ear discharge has to be differentiated from ear wax (light, dark or orange brown, normal odour) and water that entered the ear canal during shower or swimming.
- Any ear discharge that does not respond to antibiotic therapy may be caused by tuberculous OM (diagnosed by Ziehl Neelsen staining smear showing acid-fast bacilli), cholesteatoma, tumours such as rhabdomyosarcoma (see next section), and granulomatosis such as Wegener's granulomatosis. The latter one is a systemic vasculitis involving the ear, nose and throat, which manifests as otalgia, loss of hearing, tinnitus and vertigo. Diagnosis of granulomatosis is by ear inspection, tympanometry and serological and pathological studies.
- CSF otorrhoea may occur following skull fracture. Diagnosis is established by laboratory analysis showing clear fluid, which contain glucose, protein and beta 2 transferrin. The latter is diagnostic as this protein is not present in other fluids.

2. Underlying Causes of Ear Discharges
   Middle and External Ear

- Otitis externa (OE) is the most common cause of otorrhoea followed by otitis media as the second most common. In OE, otalgia predominates and usually severe
  while otorrhoea is usually scanty with absent fever. The
  pain is typically worsened by pressure on the tragus and
  the pinna. Varying degrees of conductive hearing loss
  may occur. Bacterial infection (Pseudomonas or
  Staphylococcus) accounts for the majority of cases, followed by contact dermatitis, furunculosis and herpes
  zoster infection.
- Recurrent OE may occur in children who swim with
  prolonged water exposure, so called swimmer's ear.
  Excess water in the ear keeps the ear moist and predisposing it for bacterial infection. Topical antimicrobial is
  the first line of treatment, while adding a systemic antibiotic is unlikely to be beneficial. During the acute OE
  infection, children should not swim and the ears should
  be protected.
- In OM, otorrhoea is no longer associated with otalgia
  following eardrum perforation. Culture from the discharge may grow S pneumonia, H influenzae, or Mo.

Chronic Suppurative Otitis Media (CSOM)

- CSOM is defined as a chronic inflammation of the
  middle ear and/or mastoid cavity that manifests as a
  perforation of the TM, accompanied by intermittent or
  persistent purulent discharge lasting over 2 weeks. Other
  findings include thickened granular middle ear mucosa,
  mucosal polyp and cholesteatoma. There are high levels
  of inflammatory cytokines include IL-8 that plays a significant role in the development of the chronicity.
- CSOM is differentiated from OM with effusion (OME)
  by intact TM with serous fluid.
- Culture of the discharge usually yields Pseudomonas,
  Staphylococci, or Moraxella catarrhalis.

Tympanostomy Tube Discharge

- Grommet insertion has the aim to reduce the frequency of OM and improve the hearing. Following tympanostomy tube insertion for OME at least 50% of children develop otorrhoea through the tube while the tube is properly in place.
- If the discharge occurs within 2 weeks of the tube insertion, it originates from inflammatory secretion built up in the middle ear and drains through the tube into ear canal. An ear discharge occurring after two weeks, it is most likely resulting from a new OM.
- Ear discharges from both periods usually grow non-typeable H. influenzae, S. pneumoniae, or Moraxella catarrhalis.

Tumours (Rhabdomyosarcoma)

- Rhabdomyosarcoma is the commonest types of sarcomas in children, and the majority of these tumours are localised in the neck area.
- When rhabdomyosarcoma originates from the middle ear, presenting symptoms are ear discharge, hearing loss and a mass in the external auditory canal that may resembles chronic OM. Facial palsy may occur.
- Diagnosis is established by MRI and biopsy.

Cholesteatoma

- If otorrhoea persists despite adequate antibiotic cover, cholesteatoma or rhabdomyosarcoma should be suspected.
- Cholesteatoma is a form of chronic OM. It consists of an abnormal granulomatous tissue in the middle ear cavity and mastoid process of the temporal bone. Otorrhoea results from secondary infection of this tissue. Bone erosions are very common and almost pathognomonic. Hearing loss and facial palsy are often present.
- Inspection of the tympanic membranes (TM) shows foetid otorrhoea accompanied by conductive hearing loss (findings of the acquired form), or a whitish growth behind an intact TM.

- CT scan of the ear establishes the diagnosis.

CSF Otorrhoea

- CSF leak may occur following temporal bone or skull base fractures following accidents, or occurring postoperatively following ear surgery.
- CSF leak occurs only if there is perforation of the eardrum or there is a defect in the external ear canal.
- This otogenic CSF leak is potentially life-threatening because of meningitis risk and low pressure headaches. In fact, meningitis may be the presenting problem for a child with an otologic CSF leak.
- Diagnosis of the CSF leakage is established by the presence of a clear discharge and laboratory analysis of CSF glucose, protein, and beta 2 transferrin.

Foreign Body (FB)

- Foreign body insertion into the ear is common as children, usually toddlers, are fond of inserting various items into the ear, such as beads, seeds, or toy parts. Presentation is usually with otalgia, hearing loss, or ear discharge caused by an infection of the foreign body.
- A headlamp or an illuminated magnifying glass is often required to localise and extract the FB. Its extraction by non-otolaryngologist is associated with numerous complications such as ear drum perforation and hearing loss, unless it is easily graspable.

3.4   Dizziness and Vertigo

Introduction/Core Messages
- Imbalance includes dizziness and vertigo. Dizziness is difficult to be differentiated from vertigo in young children. However, any child with possible dizziness or vertigo must be thoroughly evaluated as each can be the only symptom of a serious aetiology such as

central nervous system neoplasm or inner ear malformation.

- The most common cause of dizziness in young children is middle ear/Eustachian tube dysfunction. In older children: orthostatic hypotension = OH.
- Vertigo is not a common complaint in children in contrast to adults. While in adults, benign paroxysmal positional vertigo (BPPV) and Meniere disease are the most common causes of vertigo, in children, benign paroxysmal vertigo of childhood (BPVC), vestibular migraine and vestibular neuritis are the most common causes of vertigo.
- All children with vertigo require oto-neurological examination including search for ocular eye movements, spontaneous and positional nystagmus, caloric testing, and consideration for ear and CNS imaging.
- Unless the cause of the vertigo is clear (e.g., otitis media), close cooperation between different specialists (e.g., otologist, neurologist, ophthalmologist, and psychiatrist) is essential to establish early diagnosis and management.
- Children often cannot describe their symptoms that could lead to the correct diagnosis. Clinicians also find it difficult to differentiate the two conditions: dizziness and vertigo. For this reason diagnostic clues are provided in this section to help establish the diagnosis of each symptom.

Differential Diagnosis

Common	Rare
Otitis media and otitis media with effusion	Cerebellar tumour/acoustic neuroma
Muscular pain in the neck and shoulder area	Head injury
Orthostatic hypotension (not true vertigo)	Cholesteatoma
Benign paroxysmal vertigo of childhood	Meniere disease

Common	**Rare**
Vestibular migraine	Benign paroxysmal positional vertigo (BPPV)
Labyrinthitis/vestibular neuritis	Psychogenic
Drugs (e.g., sedative, antihistamine)	Hypoglycaemia
Epilepsy (Temporal lobe epilepsy)	Eustachian tube disease
	Epidemic vertigo (caused by a virus)

Misdiagnosis is due:

1st mistake: failing to differentiate between Dizziness from Vertigo.

2nd mistake: failing to differentiate between various causes of vertigo.

1. Diagnostic Criteria to Differentiate Between Dizziness and Vertigo

- Dizziness is a very common symptom affecting some 30–40% of older children and adolescents.
- Dizziness refers to sensation of unsteadiness without the perception that the surroundings are rotating. Orthostatic hypotension is a prototype of this category.
- As a general rule, imbalance in young children (1–5 years of age) is rarely due to dizziness, and signs of imbalance are mostly due to vertigo. Conversely, Imbalance in older children is mostly due to dizziness such as orthostatic hypotension.
- Orthostatic hypotension (OH) is characterised by reduction of systolic BP >20 mmHg within 3 min of standing or of diastolic BP >10 mmHg), which manifests as non-rotational feeling of unsteadiness or fainting when getting up from sleep or long sitting that only lasts for a minute or two but <5 min. Other symptoms include lightheadedness, nausea, sweating.

- The risk of HO is increased in dehydration or during an infectious disease.
- A young child with vertigo may not complain of vertigo but rather expressing fear and becoming pale, unsteady, and clumsy.
- In true vertigo (such as vestibular neuritis) an older child complains not only of instability, but a feeling of spinning or turning. A young child with vertigo is usually noted to appear pale and frightened and/or suddenly falling onto the ground, losing balance, stumbling or being clumsy. There is no associated hearing loss. The underlying cause is somewhere in the equilibratory pathway (eyes, semicircular canals, 8th nerve, vestibular nuclei in the brain stem).
- In case of uncertainty to differentiate between dizziness and vertigo, vestibular function is performed using audiometric examination, electronystagmography, CT or MRI scan.

2. Causes of Vertigo
   Middle Ear Disease

- Both otitis media (OM) and otitis media with effusion (OME) can cause dizziness (see above).
- Diagnosis is confirmed by symptoms and signs of OM. Audiogram and tympanometry can evaluate ear function.

   Vestibular Migraine (VM)

- VM is a common cause of episodic vertigo combining typical symptoms of migraine (a headache lasting 1–72 h, plus two of the following: bilateral or unilateral, pulsating, aggravated by routine physical activities, plus at least one of the following: nausea and or vomiting, photophobia, or phonophobia) with vestibular signs (imbalance, tinnitus, nystagmus, lasting 5 min to 72 h). Vertigo may precede or occur during or after headache. Table 3.4 summarises diagnostic criteria of VM.
- There are normal physical and neurological findings in the symptom-free intervals.

- Diagnosis is clinical and confirmed by testing the vestibular function tests (e.g., caloric response, electronystagmography, video-nystagmography, rotary chair testing) and audiogram.

Benign Paroxysmal Vertigo in Children (BPVC)

- BPVC is characterised by recurrent attacks of vertigo occurring without warning and resolving spontaneously. It is considered as a migraine precursor. Attacks occur mainly in toddlers and are usually triggered by sudden change of the head. After a few seconds there is a sudden onset of pallor, unsteadiness, crying for help, clinging to his mother or refusing to walk, often with vomiting and horizontal nystagmus. Episodes may last up to 30 s and recur in days or weeks (Table 3.5).
- Testing should include cranial nerve examination, coordination (finger-to-nose), caloric and rotational testing, and other vestibular testing such as electronystagmography.

Vestibular Neuritis (VN)/Labyrinthitis

- Both conditions have similar presentation and usually occur following a viral URTI with sudden vertigo in

TABLE 3.4 summary of diagnostic criteria of VM

- At least 5 episodes with vestibular symptoms lasting 5 min to 72 h

- Current or previous history of migraine with or without aura

- Exclusion of other causes of vestibular diseases

TABLE 3.5 Characteristic features of BPVC

- At least 5 attacks of vertigo occurring without warning that usually resolving within minutes without loss of consciousness

- There is no alternative diagnosis to explain the above symptoms

- There is no hearing loss

- Family history of migraine is common

association with nausea and vomiting. However, labyrinthitis is associated with hearing loss.

- Characteristic symptoms include sudden onset of prolonged vertigo with horizontal nystagmus, absence of auditory and neurological symptoms.
- Recovery is commonly gradual within days and weeks but imbalances may persist for months. Characteristic symptoms include sudden onset of prolonged vertigo with horizontal nystagmus, absence of auditory and neurological symptoms.
- Hearing testing (audiogram) can distinguish VN from labyrinthitis. Ice water caloric testing to confirm the abnormal vestibular function. Testing the vestibular nerve (VN) is done by holding the child in arms and rotates him or her clockwise and anticlockwise. The normal eye deviation in the direction of rotation and nystagmus in the opposite direction is absent in case of VN dysfunction.

Temporal Lobe Epilepsy (TLE)

- Any history of impaired or loss of consciousness in association with vertigo should alert the clinician that the attack could be epileptic (temporal lobe epilepsy).
- TLE is the most common cause of partial epilepsy and children often present with prodromal symptoms such as headache, irritability personal changes, and nervousness. In young child (0–3 years), motor manifestations (tonic-clonic and myoclonia) dominate the symptomatology. Older children present with dizziness, dystonic posturing, head turning, eye-mouth deviation and automatism such as lip smacking and hand clapping.
- EEG if there is a suspicion of this type of epilepsy. MRI brain scan is usually required to exclude other pathologies.

Intracranial Tumours (Acoustic neuroma)

- Tumours such as acoustic neuroma (vestibular schwannoma) are benign tumours of the cranial nerve VIII presenting with progressive unilateral hearing loss (the most common presenting symptom), tinnitus, vertigo, disequilibrium, dizziness, headache, orofacial pain, facial weakness, and abnormal gait. In contrast to vestibular neuritis and labyrinthitis, symptoms are persistent and progressive.

- Any child presenting with unremitting vertigo and nystagmus should be examined for deafness and neurological signs to exclude acoustic neuroma or cerebral degenerative disease.
- The presence of more than six café-au-lait suggests neurofibromatosis as a predisposing factor to acoustic neuroma.
- Diagnosis is established by neuro-imaging.

Further Reading

Korver AM, Smith RJH, Van Camp G, et al. Congenital hearing loss. Nat Rev Dis Primers. 2017;3:16094.

Langhagan T, Lehrer N, Borggraefe I, et al. Vestibular migraine in children and adolescents: clinical findings and laboratory tests. Front Neurol. 2014;5:292.

Olajuyin O, Olatunja OS. Aural foreign body extraction in children: a double-edged sword. Pan Afr Med J. 2015;20:186.

Venekamp RP, Javad F, van Dongen TMA, et al. Interventions for children with ear discharge occurring at least two weeks following grommet (ventilation tube) insertion. Cochrane Database Syst Rev. 2016;2016(11):CD11684.

Chapter 4
The Eye

4.1 Acutely Red Eye

Introduction/Core Messages
- Acutely red eye is common and caused by a variety of conditions including trauma such as a foreign body (FB) entering the eye, diseases of the conjunctive (conjunctivitis), cornea (keratitis), iris, ciliary body and choroid (uveitis), aqueous humour (glaucoma) and the sclera (scleritis and episcleritis).
- Clinicians should be able to diagnose most common eye diseases, which include allergic conjunctivitis (often seasonal with significant itching, runny nose, swollen lids and positive family history) and viral conjunctivitis (with its redness all over the conjunctive, watery discharge often beginning in one eye, usually caused by adenovirus).
- Any eye redness in neonates or infants requires the exclusion of nasolacrimal duct obstruction and subconjunctival haemorrhage, which may result from injury, inflammation, severe straining (e.g. in mothers during delivery), sneezing or coughing. Referral to an ophthalmologist is indicated whenever the diagnosis is unclear.

© Springer Nature Switzerland AG 2021
A. S. El-Radhi, *Avoiding Misdiagnosis in Pediatric Practice*,
In Clinical Practice, https://doi.org/10.1007/978-3-030-41750-5_4

- As red eyes can be associated with many disorders, serious underlying conditions can easily be misdiagnosed. Children and their parents may not be aware of visual impairment until late. Furthermore, children are often uncooperative for a complete ocular assessment, and inflammatory ocular changes may be too subtle to be detected. This section attempts to clarify these issues.

Differential Diagnosis

Common	Rare
Lacrimal duct obstruction	Conjunctivitis associated with systemic diseases
Viral/bacterial conjunctivitis	Acute uveitis
Chemical conjunctivitis	Dacryocystitis
Trauma (including FB)	Epidemic keratoconjunctivitis (EKC)
Allergic conjunctivitis	Cogan's syndrome (interstitial keratitis with hearing loss)
Keratitis (e.g. herpetic keratitis)	

Misdiagnosis is due to:

1st mistake: failing to differentiate common causes of acute neonatal red eyes.

2nd mistake: failing to differentiate childhood conjunctivitis from keratitis and uveitis.

1. Neonatal Red Eyes

- Episcleral and retinal haemorrhages in neonates are common after vaginal delivery. Although these seem alarming to parents and clinicians, they are harmless and disappear within 2 weeks.
- At birth, the nasolacrimal duct is often blocked. This resolves spontaneously in over 95% over the next few

months, rarely delayed until the age of 1 year and very rarely needing surgery. Diagnosis of lacrimal duct obstruction is made by the history (excessive tear production, overflow of tear onto eyelid and cheeks) and by refluxing discharge with a pressure over the lacrimal sac. Infection causes mucopurulent discharge.

- Ophthalmia neonatorum refers to inflammation of the conjunctive within the first month of life. Once principally caused by gonococcal infection, the most common cause is now chlamydia, staphylococci and chemical conjunctivitis. Ophthalmia neonatorum is a potentially blinding disease.
- Chlamydia trachomatis is the most common bacterial sexually transmitted infection worldwide. The infection can pass on to neonates by their infected mother through vertical transmission during delivery. Chlamydia infection typically occurs between 5 and 14 days after delivery. Neonates present with mucopurulent discharge with conjunctival redness and swollen eyelids. Although the infection is often harmless, untreated cases results in scarring of the cornea. In addition it can cause a serious chlamydia pneumonia in 10–20% of cases. Therefore the infection should be treated with topical and systemic antibiotics.
- Conjunctivitis in neonates may be caused by STD (sexually transmitted disease), which is acquired during vaginal delivery. Gonococcal conjunctivitis presents in the first few days of life with a profuse purulent discharge. The cornea is rapidly involved. Urgent treatment with antibiotics is required.

2. Differentiating Conjunctivitis from Keratitis/Uveitis

Conjunctival Red Eyes

- Infectious conjunctivitis (viral or bacterial) is characterised by conjunctival hyperaemia, photophobia, and ocular discharge. The palpebral involvement is typically much greater involved than the bulbar involvement (in some systemic diseases, e.g. Kawasaki disease or Lyme disease, the bulbar involvement is much greater than the palpebral one).

- The differential diagnosis between viral and bacterial conjunctivitis is easy: Viral conjunctivitis is predominantly unilateral, while bilateral conjunctivitis is more likely associated with bacterial one. In viral conjunctivitis the discharge is watery, while mucopurulent discharge predominates in bacterial one. In viral conjunctivitis, pharyngitis with pre-auricular nodes often occur; these are absent in bacterial conjunctivitis. Slit lamp examinations shows follicles in viral conjunctivitis, which is usually not present in bacterial one.
- Allergic conjunctivitis is often undiagnosed and untreated. The allergens interact with IgE to sensitise mast cells to produce histamine. Clinical symptoms are characterised by itching, redness and swelling of the conjunctiva. Corneal involvement is rare. There is often an associated atopic dermatitis and a positive history of atopy.

Non-Conjunctival Red Eyes

- Keratitis is characterised by severe ocular pain, irritation, limbus erythema, and impaired visual acuity. Cornea is swollen and may be cloudy. Worldwide, infection is an important cause of keratitis. Ocular trauma is the main predisposing factor for infection, in which corneal trauma disrupts the protective corneal epithelium, and facilitating bacterial invasion. Other predisposing factors include contact lens, prolong steroid use, facial nerve palsy and previous ocular surgery.
- Uveitis (iris, ciliary body and choroid) can be caused by infection (herpes simplex, cytomegalovirus) or non-infectious causes such as juvenile idiopathic arthritis (JIA). Clinically children present with eye redness, ocular pain, blurred or cloudy vision. Children with JIA-associated uveitis rarely express complaints, for this reason periodical eye check of JIA-patients is essential.
- Unilateral redness suggests foreign body. The latter one may need to be detected by everting the upper lid to check for concealed FB.

- Orbital cellulitis, presents as red and swollen eye, must be differentiated from rhabdomyosarcoma, which is a very aggressive malignancy of embryonic muscle tissue within the orbit. The tumour is often curable with radiation and radiotherapy.

4.2   Acute Loss of Vision

Introduction/Core Messages
- Visual loss may be acute or gradual, temporary or permanent. Acute visual loss is a frightening experience not only for children and their parents but also for the clinicians.
- Conditions causing acute visual loss in paediatrics are collectively uncommon (incidence estimated to be two–five cases per 10,000 births). It is either due to abnormalities within the ocular structure (cornea, lens, vitreous and retina) or neural visual pathways in the central nervous system (optic nerve, chiasm and cortical area).
- Although children with eye problems are often referred to ophthalmologist, clinicians should be able to perform certain eye examinations. These include examination of the visual fields (using the wiggly fingers), perform cornea light reflex, cover tests and fundoscopy. Visual acuity is tested by the child's ability to fixate and follow an object (brightly coloured toy).
- Visual loss within the eyes is easy to detect, e.g. corneal opacity, cataract or optic atrophy. Most causes of cortical visual loss occur in children with neurodisability such as asphyxia at birth, in association with seizures, spasticity or hypotonia. Rarely cortical visual loss occurs as an isolated neurological phenomenon. This section will discuss acute and transient visual loss only.

- Beware that a child with leukocoria, a white pupil, has a major clinical implication as to the likely cause is either retinoblastoma or cataract. Untreated or with delayed treatment, the retinoblastoma will lead to death, cataract to permanent vision loss.
- Detection of visual loss is essential because of availability of cure and for genetic implication (e.g. cataract, retinopathy of prematurity, glaucoma and retinoblastoma).

Differential Diagnosis

Common	Rare
Congenital visual loss	Collagen disease (e.g. rheumatoid arthritis)
Migraine	Conversion symptom (hysteria)
Amaurosis fugax	Torch infection
Raised intracranial pressure	Acute glaucoma
Optic neuritis	
Occipital lobe seizures	
Drugs (e.g. steroid)	

Misdiagnosis is due to:
1st mistake: inability to detect visual loss early.
2nd mistake: failing to detect important causes of visual loss.

1. Early Detection of Visual Loss

- Eye examination is an essential part of neonatal examination, including using the ophthalmoscope held at a distance of 20–25 cm to look for the red reflex. This is usually done on the third day. Fundoscopy is usually unnecessary.
- In ophthalmology, more than in any other specialty, observation is the most important technique to detect abnormalities. Get the child interested and assess his/

her ability to fixate and follow a target such as bright-red object or the light source of a torch. This can be performed by the age of about 6 weeks.

- For school age, E-test is used whereby a child points in the direction of the letter. Later Snellen acuity charts are used for the age group 5 or 6 years.

2. Important Causes of Visual Loss (see also Section of Red Eye above)

Migraine (see also Section of Headaches)

- Visual symptoms are common in migraine, either in the form of aura or photophobia. The aura phenomenon is linked to cortical alterations localised in the visual cortex; photophobia is linked to thalamic structures.
- The most common cause for transient visual loss in children occurs during a visual aura of a classic migraine. Aura is defined by the International Headache Society as a recurrent disorder that develops over 5–29 min and lasts for <1 h.

Amaurosis Fugax

- Transient monocular lasting 1–5 min is usually referred to as amaurosis fugax resulting from cerebral ischemia (seizure, stroke). While migraine aura may present with flashes of light (photopsia), amaurosis fugax presents as blackout of vision or a curtain across the vision.
- The painless transient loss of vision is a direct result from interruption of blood supply to the retina which shows signs of ischaemia. Causes include emboli, ipsilateral internal carotid artery occlusion of stenosis. Predisposing conditions to amaurosis fugax include polycythaemia, sickle cell anaemia and homocystinuria.
- Predisposing conditions to amaurosis fugax include polycythaemia, sickle-cell anaemia, homocystinuria.

Optic Neuritis (Multiple Sclerosis)

- Patient with optic neuritis usually presents with pain on eye movement in one eye, in addition to visual loss. Pupillary light reflex is weaker in the affected eye, and the optic disc is mildly oedematous.

TABLE 4.1 Differences between paediatric and adult MS

• MS in children affects both sexes, while adult MS affects more female than male
• Paediatric MS has more intracranial demyelinating process and axonal damage compared to adults
• Paediatric MS has more relapse rate leading to early disability than in adults
• MRI: early brain atrophy (compared to adults) and hypodense focal lesions

- Causes of optic neuritis in children include multiple sclerosis (MS), steroid medication and acute disseminated encephalomyelitis.
- Children with MS present with visual problems, inability to walk and cognitive and neuro-psychiatric deficits.
- Although most cases of optic neuritis in adults are due to MS, this is uncommon but increasingly recognised in paediatric population. Differences between paediatric and adult MS are shown in Table 4.1.

Increased Intracranial Pressure (ICP)

- In contrast to optic neuritis, visual loss is an unusual presenting symptom in children who usually present with headaches, vomiting, cranial nerve palsies and personality-behavioural changes.
- Idiopathic intracranial hypertension=IIH (previously termed pseudo-tumour cerebri, or benign intracranial hypertension) is often associated with visual impairment. Characteristic features of IIH include papilloedema, normal cerebral imaging and increased CSF pressure on LP.

Occipital Lobe Seizures (OLS)

- Occipital seizures (such as benign partial epilepsy with occipital paroxysm) are not rare; visual symptoms are prominent and include amaurosis, multi-coloured illusions or hallucinations and eye deviation, followed by hemiclonic seizures or automatisms.

- OLS occurs mostly during sleep or on awakening. EEG is usually diagnostic: spike-waves are seen uni-or bilaterally in the occipital region on eye closure.

Glaucoma

Congenital glaucoma manifests as large eye ball, epiphora (overflow of tears), photophobia, blepharospasm and hazy or red eye, and confirmed by raised intraocular pressure.

Nystagmus

This fro-and-to oscillation of the eye results from an abnormality at some point in the visual pathway. It is commonly associated with conditions with congenital poor vision including corneal opacity and retinopathy of prematurity. Acquired nystagmus occurs in association with intracranial space-occupying lesion, metabolic and degenerative CNS disorders.

Drugs

- Numerous drugs may cause optic neuropathy include anti-convulsants (e.g. Vigabatrin, Ethambutol, Amiodarone).
- Some systemically administered medications, e.g. steroids, may cause cataract. Steroids may also cause glaucoma.

4.3   Double Vision (Diplopia)

Introduction/Core Messages
- Diplopia, simultaneous perception of two images of a single object, is less common in children than in adults because of the lower incidence of strokes and other intracranial lesions.
- The most common cause of diplopia in children is misalignment of the visual axes occurring particularly in disorders affecting the cranial nerves (third, fourth and sixth) innervating the six ocular muscles. Other

causes involve mechanical interference with ocular motion or disorder of neuromuscular transmission.

- Diplopia is either binocular (true diplopia) or monocular. The latter is caused by abnormality in the cornea (e.g. severe astigmatism = irregular curvature), in the lens (e.g. cataract, dislocated lens) or in the vitreous humour (e.g. vitreous cysts).

- Diplopia is often the first manifestation of many systemic muscular or neurologic disorders, some of which are of a serious nature. Therefore, prompt evaluation is usually required. A detailed history and examination will make it possible to determine which muscles and ocular nerves are affected and what is the likely cause.

- Although diplopia does occur in infants, they do not usually present with diplopia and therefore the causes in infants are not included in this section.

Differential Diagnosis

Common	Rare
Physiological	Myasthenia gravis
Strabismus (particularly paralytic)	Drugs (e.g. anti-epileptics)
Post-surgery for refractive errors	Increased intracranial pressure (ICP)
Ophthalmoplegic migraine	Möbius' syndrome
3rd, 4th or 6th cranial nerve palsy	Thyroid ophthalmoplegia

Misdiagnosis is due to:

1st mistake: failing to detect early symptoms and signs of diplopia.

2nd mistake: failing to differentiate causes of diplopia.

1. Early Detection of Diplopia in Children

- The most common cause of diplopia is strabismus. However the brain of a young child learns how to suppress the image of the weaker, misaligned eye. Therefore, diplopia is usually not the presenting complaint in young age. Presentation may be with squint, covering one eye with one hand or tilting the head to one side.

- Differentiating monocular from binocular diplopia is simple: covering each eye will correct diplopia in binocular, while diplopia persists in the monocular of the affected eye.
- Ophthalmoplegic migraine presents as third-nerve palsy ipsilateral to the hemicranial of the headache due to vasoconstriction during the attack to this nerve.
- Diplopia may be the first complaint in children with dislocated lens occurring in conditions such Marfan's syndrome (excessive height, dilated aortic route) and homocystinuria (malar flush, neurodisability, thrombo-embolic events).
- Although diplopia is a common symptom in posterior fossa tumour, children rarely complain of it, as they are able to suppress the image of the affected eye. Instead, head tilting may occur as this position is an attempt to align the two images.
- Typically, a fourth nerve palsy manifests with head tilting opposite to the affected eye, while sixth-nerve palsy tilts toward the palsied nerve.
- Although the diagnosis of diplopia caused by ocular muscle palsy is fairly easy, a final diagnosis is unlikely to be reached at primary setting. Referral to an ophthalmologist is usually required.
- A typical basilar artery migraine should be differentiated from intracranial tumour that causes similar symptoms. An urgent CT scan or MRI is often needed, particularly if it is the first episode.
- When a child presents with diplopia and ptosis, third-nerve palsy is likely. However, Horner's syndrome is another possibility. Small pupil and reduced sweating on the affected side will help to differentiate both conditions.
- The sixth nerve has a long intracranial course so it is susceptible to damage from cranial tumour. An acquired sixth-nerve palsy is usually an ominous sign requiring immediate attention. Adolescents with hysteria may present with diplopia; this diagnosis should be one of exclusion.

2. Causes of Diplopia

Diplopia can arise from one eye (monocular) or may occur when the eyes are misaligned (binocular). Types of diplopia include horizontal, vertical and oblique diplopia.

Monocular Diplopia

- Cases of monocular are infrequent (compared to binocular), mostly benign, and usually caused by intraocular pathology such as incurred refractive error, lesions of the cornea (astigmatism), lens (cataract, dislocated lens) or iris (iridocyclitis).
- The diplopia persists when 1 eye is closed.

Binocular Diplopia

- This is more frequent than monocular diplopia. The diplopia disappears when 1 eye is closed.
- The main cause of diplopia is a misalignment of the visual axis. Other causes include congenital myopathies, palsies of the 3rd, 4th and 6th cranial nerve (tumour, neurodegenerative diseases) and drugs (botulinum toxin, anticonvulsants such as Gabapentin and Topiramate).
- Myasthenia gravis (MG) is a very important cause of diplopia. MG is an autoimmune disease characterised by fatigability and muscle weakness. Ocular muscles are predominately affected with ptosis and diplopia as the most common presenting clinical features.

4.4   Squint (Strabismus)

Introduction/Core Messages
- Strabismus or squint, misalignment of the eyes, is a common ophthalmic problem, affecting 4–5% of children younger than 6 years of age. Strabismus is diagnosed clinically, which involves examination of the corneal light reflex and cover test.

- Strabismus may be transient or constant, manifest or latent. Because of different causes and treatments, it is important to divide strabismus into non-paralytic and paralytic.
- Risk factors of having squint include prematurity (retinopathy of prematurity), genetic influence, maternal smoking during pregnancy, and surgery for cataract. Untreated squint results in loss of binocular vision, amblyopia, impact on psychosocial wellbeing such as low self-esteem and interaction with peers, poor school performance and employment prospect.
- Strabismus should never be ignored; it is never outgrown.
- In a child with any ocular disorder, particularly squint, assessment of the visual acuity, is essential.
- Amblyopia (lazy eye) is a reduction of visual acuity of one or both eyes caused by poor visual stimulation early in life subsequent to conditions such as strabismus, congenital cataract, or optic atrophy.

Differential Diagnosis

Common	Rare
• Pseudo-strabismus	Parinaud's syndrome
• Congenital (infantile) strabismus	Migraine ophthalmoplegia
• Intermittent strabismus	Möbius' syndrome (congenital bilateral facial weakness)
• Paralytic strabismus	Duane's syndrome (congenital impaired eye motility)
• Accommodation strabismus	Parinaud's syndrome (congenital weakness in vertical gaze)

Misdiagnosis is due to:

1st mistake: difficulty in detecting squint clinically.

2nd mistake: failing to distinguish untrue (pseudo-squint) from true squint.

3rd mistake: failing to differentiate non-paralytic squint and paralytic squint.

1. How to Diagnose Squint?

- Gross strabismus is usually noticed by members of the family or carers.
- Eye movements: Child is asked to (or attracted to) look at an object/toy which is moved in different directions at around 30 cm. Paralytic squint can easily be detected.
- Corneal light reflex: Useful for children who are not cooperative (below the age of 3 years). A light source is held between the examiner and the child at 25 cm. The light reflection is seen in the centre of the child's pupil in healthy eyes and in children with pseudo-squint.
- Cover test is based on the observation of a re-fixation movement of a deviated eye when the fixing eye is covered, while the child looks at a distant object of 3 m. This establishes the diagnosis of manifest strabismus. The presence of latent strabismus is assessed by using the alternate cover test: Re-fixation movements occur in either eyes as the cover is removed. If no movement occurs, there is no strabismus.
- Prism alternate cover test is used for ocular alignment measurements.

2. Features of Pseudo-Squint

- Up to the age of 6 months, intermittent strabismus is a normal developmental milestone, occurring particularly as outward deviation in about two-thirds of neonates. After the age of 6 months, any degree of strabismus needs to be evaluated.
- Pseudo-strabismus = false appearance of squint in normal eyes is a common cause of referral to ophthalmologist. The normal alignment can be shown by the normal corneal light reflexes. There is also no re-fixation movement when the cover test is used.

- Epicanthic folds are folds across the inner corner of the eyes (canthus), usually from the upper lids or caused by broad flat nasal bridge. Epicanthic folds are present in most infants and young children and become less apparent later, coinciding with peaking of the nasal bridge. If theses folds are prominent, they give the impression of pseudo-strabismus.

3. Distinguishing Non-Paralytic from Paralytic Squint
   Characteristics of Non-Paralytic Strabismus

- This type of strabismus is usually congenital. It may only be noticed when the child is tired.
- Non-paralytic or concomitant strabismus includes inward deviation of the eyes (esophorias, commonly known as convergent or inward or crossed eyes), outward deviation of the eyes (known as exophorias, or divergent strabismus) and hyper-deviation (upward) and hypo-deviation (downward) deviation of an eye.
- Both eyes have full movements in all directions of gaze when tested separately.
- Double vision (diplopia) does not occur, but the eye that does not fixate usually has amblyopia.

Characteristics of Paralytic Strabismus

- Paralytic strabismus involves palsy of the third, fourth or sixth cranial nerve. It is usually acquired. The corneal light reflex is normal in paralytic strabismus.
- Diagnosis can be suggested by the two symptoms of head tilting and double vision that increases when the eye is moving in the direction of the paralytic muscle. Characteristically, a child with diplopia compensate by closing the eyelid of the paralytic eye. Tilting of the head occurs to the position of the better eye.
- A fourth ocular nerve palsy causes a contralateral head tilt, i.e. a head tilt to the right caused by a left-sided nerve palsy and vice versa. Conversely, a sixth-nerve palsy causes head tilting on the same side of the palsy. The reason for the tilt is to avoid diplopia.

- Retinoblastoma, with an incidence of one in 20,000 births, is the most important cause of acquired strabismus, affecting children younger than 5 years of age in 95% of cases. The tumour is initiated by mutation of the retinoblastoma gene (RB1). Children usually present with unilateral leukocoria (white pupil) as the most common presenting sign, followed by strabismus, orbital inflammation and a red eye reflex (cat eye). The tumour is curable if diagnosed and treated early, but death is inevitable if untreated.

4.5   Proptosis (Exophthalmos)

Introduction/Core Messages
- Proptosis, exophthalmos or protrusion of the eyes, is a forward displacement of the eye, which may be caused by a congenital shallow orbit (craniofacial malformation such as oxycephaly, Crouzon's syndrome), trauma (orbital haemorrhage), inflammation (orbital cellulitis, abscess), vascular diseases (e.g. haemangioma, cavernous sinus thrombosis), central nervous system anomaly (encephalocele), endocrine (e.g. Graves' disease) or neoplasms (optic glioma, meningioma, metastatic neuroblastoma).
- Posterior displacement of the eye is termed enophthalmos that may occur following atrophy of the orbital tissue in cases with severe dehydration.
- A proptotic eye not adequately protected by the lids is at risk of keratopathy, strabismus, diplopia, optic nerve atrophy and decreased visual acuity. Urgent management is required.
- A case of proptosis in a child requires the presence of a multidisciplinary team with collaboration of differential specialties including ophthalmology, neurosurgery, oncology, radiotherapy and otorhinolaryngology.

Differential Diagnosis

Common	**Rare**
Shallow orbit (e.g. Crouzon's syndrome)	Plexiform neurofibroma
Orbital tumours	Graves's disease
Retinoblastoma	Meningioma (involving the sphenoid wing)
Leukaemia	Sarcoidosis
Haemangioma	Orbital encephalocele
Teratoma	Histiocytosis X
Metastatic neuroblastoma	
Paranasal sinusitis	
Orbital cellulitis	

Misdiagnosis is due to:

1st mistake: ignoring the earliest symptoms and signs of proptosis in children.

2nd mistake: ignoring that systemic diseases may often present as unilateral proptosis.

1. Early Symptoms and Signs of Proptosis

- Early symptoms and signs of proptosis include eye pain, irritability, lacrimation, visual disturbance and restriction of eye movements, diplopia, and chemosis (swelling or oedema of the conjunctiva).
- Clinician faced with a child with proptosis should be able to do ophthalmic examination to diagnose proptosis and the likely cause, including assessment of visual acuity, ocular muscle movement, measuring of proptosis, pupillary size and reaction to light, fundi and performing systemic examination.
- The proptosis can be measured by exophthalmometry, which measures the distance between the lateral angle of the bony orbit and the cornea (normal values for adults <20 mm). Generally, a distance of 2mm or greater asymmetry between the protrusion of the two eyes is considered abnormal.

2. Unilateral and Bilateral Proptosis

- The differentiating between unilateral and bilateral causes of proptosis is very useful in order to narrow the differential diagnosis. Retro-orbital tumours such as haemangioma and dermoid cyst usually cause unilateral proptosis.
- As shown on Table 4.2, systemic diseases such as Graves' disease, leukaemia and lymphoma may present as unilateral or bilateral proptosis.
- Orbital capillary haemangioma (rarely cavernous haemangioma) is the most common space-occupying tumour in children that is often found behind the eye globe causing painless proptosis. The natural history of haemangioma is a rapid growth during the first 6 months of life and regresses spontaneously when the child reaches 4–6 years of age.
- Optic gliomas are very common with neurofibromatosis typ1, NF-1 (15%). They are usually benign and asymptomatic, and commonly present with visual disturbance, visual field defects, nystagmus, strabismus and optic disc pallor on fundoscopy.
- Neuroblastoma, the most common solid tumour of childhood, metastasises frequently into the orbit causing unilateral periorbital ecchymosis in addition to

TABLE 4.2 Causes of unilateral and bilateral proptosis

Unilateral	Bilateral
Graves' disease	Graves' disease
Haemangioma	Crouzon's syndrome
Leukaemia	Leukaemia
Lymphoma (non-Hodgkin's)	Lymphoma (non-Hodgkin's)
Orbital cellulitis/paranasal sinusitis	
Neuroblastoma/rhabdomyosarcoma	
Dermoid cyst	
Lymphangioma	

proptosis. The tumour may arise from the adrenals, cervical sympathetic chain or mediastinum. Orbital rhabdomyosarcoma is the most common soft tissue sarcoma in children presenting as rapidly progressing proptosis often misdiagnosed as orbital cellulitis.

4.6 Eyelid Disorders and Ptosis (Blepharoptosis)

Introduction/Core Messages
- Eyelid disorders are exceedingly common in children and range from benign, self-resolving to serious malignant or metastatic processes.
- Two separate muscles are involved in the elevation of the eyelid: the superior levator palpebrae (innervated by 3rd cranial nerve) and the superior tarsal muscle (innervated by cervical sympathetic system).
- The diagnosis of any eyelid abnormality, including ptosis, requires thorough systemic examination and sometimes investigations, to confirm the cause of this abnormality.
- Children with ptosis (drooping of the upper eyelid) commonly raise the eyebrows or lift the chin to maintain binocular vision.
- Children with ptosis should be referred for ophthalmic opinion, particularly if they have abnormal head posture, amblyopia, abnormal visual field and it is cosmetically unacceptable.

Differential Diagnosis

Common	Rare
Coloboma	Marcus Gunn jaw-winking phenomenon
Horner's syndrome	Meibomian cyst
Congenital ptosis	Muscular dystrophy (facio-scapulo-humeral)

Common	**Rare**
Acquired ptosis	Myotonic muscular dystrophy
Congenital ectropion/ entropion	
Myasthenia gravis	
Infection of the eyelids blepharitis	
Chalazion (inflammation)	
Acute blepharitis	

Misdiagnosis is due to:

1st mistake: not recognising common abnormalities affecting the eyelids.

2nd mistake: failing to distinguish benign from serious causes of ptosis.

3rd mistake: not recognising signs of Horner's syndrome

1. Common Abnormalities of the Eyelids

- Coloboma is a defect or a hole (usually oval in shape) affecting one structure of the eye (e.g. eye lid, iris, retina) that may be associated with other abnormalities such as cataract or glaucoma.
- Entropion (Trichiasis or ingrowing eyelashes) can be congenital caused by orbicularis muscle hypertrophy, or spasm of the muscle, or acquired due to scarring or infection, particularly trachoma.
- Patients with ectropion (outward-turning of the lid margin) are at risk of exposure keratopathy, overflow of tears and conjunctivitis. This may occur in association with facial palsy resulting from weakness of the orbicularis muscle. Urgent ophthalmic consultation is required.
- Eyebrow abnormalities include sparse or absent eyebrows (e.g. alopecia, ectodermal dysplasia) and eyebrows joining together medially (Waardenburg's syndrome, Cornelia de Lang syndrome).

2. Benign and Serious Causes of Ptosis
   Benign Causes of Ptosis

- Congenital ptosis is usually due to absent of the ocular superior levator muscle or dysfunctional innervation by the superior branch of the 3rd cranial nerve and the superior tarsal muscle, which is innervated by the cervical sympathetic system.
- In Marcus Gunn jaw-winking (5% of all cases with ptosis), the upper lid rises as the jaw opens. This is caused by synkinesis between the third and fifth cranial nerves.
- Children with Bell's palsy usually present acutely with facial nerve palsy as an isolated entity without involvement of other cranial nerve or brainstem dysfunction. Symptoms also include difficulty in closing and opening eyelid, impaired taste and excessive tearing.
- Ophthalmoplegic migraine may involve the 3rd nerve causing ptosis.
- Horner's syndrome (HS): resulting from disruption of the sympathetic nervous system and is characterised by a triad of ipsilateral ptosis, ocular miosis causing anisocoria (unequal size of the eye pupils). Benign causes of HS are birth trauma and post-viral nerve damage (see HS below).
- Duane retraction syndrome is a congenital ocular movement disorder associated with limitation of horizontal eye movements in addition to ptosis. The syndrome is due to hypoplasia or absence of the 6th cranial nerve.

   Serious Causes of Ptosis

- Myasthenia Gravis (MG)

  - MG is a heterogeneous group of disorders affecting neuromuscular transmission. It is an autoimmune disease caused by antibodies against the neurotransmitter acetylcholine.
  - Typical presentation is muscle fatigue that worsens after a period of physical activity and improves after

periods of rest. Muscles involved are those of the eyes (ptosis causing diplopia), face and swallowing.

- Diagnosis is made by detection antibodies against acetylcholine receptors, and confirmed by edrophonium (Tensilon) test.

- Other serious causes include neuropathic disorders (e.g. 3rd nerve palsy due to intracranial tumour), myopathic disorders (e.g. limb-girdle muscular dystrophy, myotonic dystrophy, oculo-pharyngeal muscular dystrophy).

3. Horner's Syndrome (HS)

- HS consists of unilateral ptosis, ipsilateral miosis and facial anhidrosis with preserved pupil reaction to light. HS results from ipsilateral oculo-sympathetic pathway.
- In children, HS may be the first sign of an occult malignancy such as mediastinal tumour in the form of neuroblastoma in otherwise asymptomatic individuals. Neuroblastoma is the most common occult malignancy associated.
- The appearance of HS warrants prompt investigation including urinary catecholamines and imaging of the head, neck and thorax.

Further Reading

Borchert M, Liu GT, Pineles S, et al. Pediatric optic neuritis: what is new? J Neuroophthamol. 2017;37(Suppl 1):S14–22. https://doi.org/10.1097/wno.0000000000000551.

Chawla R, Kellner JD, Astle WF. Acute infectious conjunctivitis in children. Pediatr Child Health. 2001;6(6):329–35.

Cotter S, Varma R, Tarczy-Hornoch K, et al. Risk factors associated with childhood strabismus. Ophthalmology. 2011;118(11):2251–61.

Chapter 5
The Neck

5.1 Neck Lumps (Lymphadenopathy)

Introduction/Core Messages

- Human body has about 600 lymphnodes. They act as a filter between lymphatic and haematological circulations. They contain immunological cells including macrophages, B and T-cells. Some lymphnodes are present in virtually every child; total absence of palpable lymphnodes suggests the possibility of immune deficiency such as agammaglobulinaemia.
- About one-third of neonates have palpable lymphnodes, usually smaller than 1 cm in diameter. They are commonly present in the inguinal area due to infection of the nappy area.
- Although the most common cause of cervical lumps is benign reactive lymphadenitis caused by a viral upper respiratory tract infection, other neck masses are common in children and might be mistaken as enlarged lymphnodes.
- Generalised lymphadenopathy indicates involvement of enlarged lymphnodes in two or more than two node regions. Generalised lymphadenopathy

© Springer Nature Switzerland AG 2021
A. S. El-Radhi, *Avoiding Misdiagnosis in Pediatric Practice*,
In Clinical Practice, https://doi.org/10.1007/978-3-030-41750-5_5

suggests either systemic infection (e.g. viral such as Epstein–Barr, AIDS, mononucleosis or toxoplasmosis), autoimmune disease (e.g. JIA, SLE) or malignancy (e.g. leukaemia, lymphoma).

- Although most cases of lymphadenopathy are benign, diagnosis in unexplained cases cannot be ascertained on clinical grounds alone. Autoimmune diseases, leukaemia, lymphoma, mycobacterium lymphadenitis, and medications need to be considered in the differential diagnosis. Imaging and tissue biopsy are essential to clarify the diagnosis.

Differential Diagnosis

Common	Rare
Reactive lymphadenitis due to local infection	Cystic hygroma
Goitre	Juvenile idiopathic arthritis
Systemic infection (e.g. mononucleosis, HIV)	Branchial cyst
Sternomastoid tumour	Cat-scratch fever
Dermoid cyst/lipoma	Systemic lupus erythematosus
Malignancy (e.g. Lymphoma, rhabdomyosarcoma)	Drugs (e.g. INH, phenytoin)
Thyroglossal cyst	
TB lymphadenitis	

Misdiagnosis is due to:

1st mistake: lack of basic knowledge about lymphadenopathy.

2nd mistake: failing to differentiate inflammatory causes of lymphadenopathy.

3rd mistake: failing to differentiate non-inflammatory causes of lymphadenopathy.

4th mistake: difficulty in establishing the diagnosis of malignant lymphadenopathy.

1. Basic Knowledge of Lymphadenopathy (Tables 5.1 and 5.2)

- Approximately 40% of the total lymphnodes of the human body are in the cervical region, normally <1 cm in diameter. They are usually detectable in children aged 3–5 years of age, reached their largest diameter around the age 4–8 years in over 90%, followed by gradual regress after adolescence. These lymphnodes in the neck are usually benign reactive lymphnode enlargement resulting from lymphadenitis and caused by viral infections in the upper airway, leaving small (<1 cm), non-tender, mobile lymphnodes that are considered normal in children.

- Cervical lymphnodes drain lymph from the head and neck areas; submental and submandibular lymphnodes drain from the buccal mucosa, cheek and nose; supra-clavicular lymphnodes drain from right-sided thorax

TABLE 5.1 Clinical features of lymphadenopathy

• Location	Whether localised or generalised will narrow the differential diagnosis
• Size	<1 cm or >1 cm
• Pain/tenderness	Suggests infection
• Consistency	Firm-to-hard consistency suggests chronic inflammation caused fibrotic changes. Hard and painless lymphnode suggests TB infection or tumour
• Mobility	Freely movable suggests infection or collagen disease. Matted together lymphnode suggests TB infection, sarcoidosis or lymphoma
• Organomegaly	Splenomegaly suggests infections (such as mononucleosis) or lymphoma
• Systemic signs	Suggest infections such as mononucleosis or malignancy

TABLE 5.2 Lymphnode diseases according to lymphnode localisation

• Cervical	Viral benign reactive
	Bacterial (staphylococcal, streptococcal, cat-scratch fever, TB)
	Malignancy (lymphoma)
• Supraclavicular	Abdominal or thoracic malignancy, tuberculosis
• Axillary	Viral non-specific reactive
	Bacterial (staphylococcal, streptococcal)
	Cat-scratch fever
• Inguinal	Benign reactive to viral infection, rash in the nappy area
	Malignancy

and left-sided abdomen; axillary drain from the ipsilateral arm, breast and neck; and inguinal lymphnodes drain from the ipsilateral leg and buttocks.

- Lymphadenopathy indicates abnormalities in the size, consistency and/or number of lymphnodes. Pathological lymphadenopathy that requires immediate attention includes large lymphnodes (diameter exceeds 1 cm for cervical and axillary, and 1.5 cm for inguinal lymphnodes, tender, matted together or fixed to the skin or underlying structures, or localised in the supraclavicular area. Palpable supraclavicular lymphnodes of any size are abnormal.

2. Inflammatory/Infectious Lumps at the Neck

Inflammatory lymphadenopathy includes viral and bacterial lymphadenitis, autoimmune diseases, and malignancies, and medications.

- Viral Lymphadenitis

Of the many lumps found in the neck, viral lymphadenitis is the most common and important physical finding. It usually caused by viral infections (e.g. rhinovirus, Epstein-Barr, respiratory syncytial virus), leading to multiple, small (<1 cm in diameter), usually bilateral, non-tender, firm and mobile lymphnodes, which are so common that they can be considered normal in children. Cervical lymphadenopathy usually refers to cervical lymphnodes measuring >1 cm in diameter.

- Bacterial Lymphadenitis

  - Bacterial lymphadenitis is defined as an acute lymphadenitis that improves (particularly fever) on antibiotics, or bacteria can be identified by culture through aspiration or surgical means.
  - Classical presentation is enlarged and tender lymphnodes, overlying skin erythema with systemic manifestations such as fever, anorexia and pain at the neck.
  - Toxoplasma gondii, a protozoan parasites, can cause chronic posterior cervical lymphadenitis as the most common form of an acquired toxoplasmosis.

- Granulomatous Disease (TB, Sarcoidosis)

  - The predominant cause of tuberculous adenopathy in the tropics is in cervical region in over 90% of cases, affecting mostly submandibular or submental region. Lymphnodes are matted, firm, and immobile on palpation. Clinical signs include malaise, low-grade fever and night sweats.
  - In developed countries, systemic features are usually lacking, chest X-ray normal, Mantoux test often negative, and anti-tuberculous drugs are ineffective. Non-tuberculous mycobacterial bacilli, most commonly Mycobacterium avium, cause lymphadenitis that is acquired through oral cavity and manifests as chronic granulomatous lymphadenopathy. It is cured by excision of the affected lymphnode.
  - Biopsy of a lymphnode shows granulomatous tissue with central caseous necrosis. Needle aspiration has the risk of causing a fistula.
  - Sarcoidosis is multi-system disease characterised in younger children (< 6 years) by uveitis, skin rash and arthritis, Older children present with hilar lymphadenopathy and pulmonary symptoms.

- HIV Infection
  - Cervical lymphadenopathy is often among the initial presentation in HIV infected patients. The presence of oral candida or gingivitis supports the diagnosis.
  - Diagnosis is established by laboratory means.
- Kawasaki Disease (KD) (see also the Section of pharyngo-tonsillitis).
  - KD may present with fever and cervical lymphadenopathy only causing difficulty to differentiate it from bacterial lymphadenitis before other KD symptoms appear late. Delaying diagnosis and treatment of KD lymphadenitis can lead to serious cardiac complications.
  - Diagnosis of KD lymphadenitis can be suspected when antibiotic treatment shows no effect on the fever. KD lymphadenitis shows no evidence of abscess formation in contrast to bacterial lymphadenitis.
- Cat-Scratch Fever (CSF)
  - Following licking, scratching or biting by a kitten, a papule develops at the site of inoculation about a week later. Regional lymphadenitis is noted within few weeks later in about 90% that undergo spontaneous resolution within 2–4 months. Some patients experience malaise, mild fever and anorexia.
  - Other uncommon presentation includes PUO, hepatosplenic granuloma and osteomyelitis.
  - Serological testing identifies antibody to B henselae bacteria. Aspiration and using Warthin–Starry sliver stain suggest the diagnosis. MRI or CT-scan has little diagnostic value.
- Mononucleosis (see Section Pharyngo-tonsillitis).

3. Non-Inflammatory Lumps at the Neck

- Thyroglossal Cyst
  - The cyst develops from remnant thyroglossal duct, which is painless but becomes enlarged and tender if infected.

- Pathognomonic sign is a midline position and its vertical movement on swallowing and tongue protrusion. About 10% arises under the chin and present as submental swelling. These cysts are the second most common neck masses after lymphnodes.
- A thyroglossal cyst should never be excised unless a thyroid tissue is excluded.

- Sternomastoid Tumour

  - This mass is usually caused by overstretching and myolysis of the sternomastoid muscle during a difficult delivery.
  - The mass is usually detected few weeks after birth as a lump in the third of the sternomastoid muscle. It can cause shortening of the muscle and wry neck (torticollis) with the face looking away from the affected side.

- Branchial Cyst

  - The cyst looks like an insignificant papule on the side of the neck, off centre (in contrast to thyroglossal cyst), anterior to the middle third of the sternomastoid muscle. It often becomes prominent after an upper respiratory tract infection.
  - These cysts are remnant from branchial arches which are well developed ridges of the embryo from 4 to 8 week of gestation. Its surgical removal may be quite difficult to trace out its tract.

- Goitre

  - Thyroid disorders are one of the most common endocrine disorders manifesting as various pathologies (Table 5.3). The most common presentation is a diffuse enlargement of the thyroid gland (goitre) with or without hormonal deficiency or excess.
  - Defects in thyroid hormone synthesis (dyshormonogenesis) occur mostly in the neonatal period as congenital goitre (15–20% of the neonates with an abnormal screening test.
  - The most common acquired goitre in children is chronic lymphocytic thyroiditis (Hashimoto thyroid-

TABLE 5.3 Short list of common causes of goitre in children

- Dyshormonogenesis
- Simple goitre
- Autoimmune thyroid diseases
  - Chronic lymphocytic thyroiditis (Hashimoto's)
  - Graves
- Infection
  - Subacute viral thyroiditis
  - Bacterial thyroiditis
- Anatomic abnormalities
  - Thyroglossal duct cyst
  - Nodular goitre, e.g. solitary nodule or cancer

itis), accounting for 55–65% of euthyroid goitre. Hypothyroidism may occur.

- Autoimmune Diseases
  - Juvenile idiopathic arthritis, JIA, often presents with generalised lymphadenopathy, seen mostly in systemic form (Still's disease) in association with fever, rash (salmon-pink) and hepatosplenomegaly.
  - Systemic lupus erythematosus, SLE, involves multi-organs including malar rash, nephropathy, arthritis.
  - Painless generalised lymphadenopathy may precede the other symptoms of SLE by months and years. Screening for SLE in an unexplained lymphadenopathy can clinch the diagnosis.

4. Characteristic Features of Malignant Lymphadenopathy

- Characteristic signs of malignant lymphadenopathy are rubbery and fixed lymphnodes, which are usually bilateral, non-tender and without any skin changes. Associated systemic manifestations include fever, weight loss and night sweating.
- Although the prevalence of malignancy is low (less than 1% of all causes of lymphadenopathy), the presence of

lymphnodes remains a significant source of concern for both parents and professionals. The rate of malignancies rises sharply with age. In paediatric setting, most malignant diagnoses include lymphoma, rhabdomyosarcoma and neuroblastoma.

- Referral to an oncology specialist is particularly indicated and urgent as diagnostic delay will cause poor delays: if the lymphnodes are matted or fixed, >2 cm in diameter, matted together, hard in consistency, grows rapidly within two weeks and does not show shrinkage or regress within the following weeks, or associated with persistent or unexplained fever, night sweat, or anorexia or weight loss.
- Lymphnodes localised at the supraclavicular region should always be carefully evaluated for possible malignancy.
- Ultrasound scan should be the first tool of examination as this can assess the number, size, pattern of vascularity and internal structure of the lymphnodes. Findings for possible malignancy include absence of hilum and undetectable cortical and medullary contours. Fine needle aspiration has a high specificity and sensitivity, particularly if the procedure is guided by endoscopic ultrasonography, is less invasive, cheaper and quicker to perform. Elevated CRP and lactate dehydrogenase, and leukopenia support the aetiology of lymphoma, while pancytopenia and the presence of blast cells support leukaemia.

5.2   Stiff/Tilt Neck (Meningism and Meningitis)

Introduction/Core Messages
- Neck stiffness is a common complaint in paediatrics to both emergency and primary care services. The term refers to abnormal position of the neck or restricted range of movement, usually associated with pain during passive and active movements.

Of the many causes of stiff neck, the most important cause is meningitis. Other causes include muscle spasm (strain or sprain), polymyalgia, arthritis (ankylosing spondylitis) and cervical spine abnormalities.

- Meningism indicates resistance to neck flexion due to meningeal irritation without intracranial inflammation. Symptoms are similar to those of meningitis, which include headache, photophobia and vomiting. Causes include febrile viral or bacterial infection, such as pneumonia, or adverse reaction to drugs such as (rarely) NSAIDs (non-steroidal anti-inflammatory drugs). Spinal fluid pressure is often elevated but spinal fluid is otherwise normal. In contrast to torticollis, a child with meningism is usually ill looking with fever. CSF examination is usually required to exclude meningitis.

- This symptom of meningism is extremely important because of the possibility of meningitis. When a child presents with fever, headache and photophobia, CNS infection should be excluded as a matter of urgency.

Differential Diagnosis

Common	Rare
Meningitis, meningococcal disease (MCD)	Visual defects (nystagmus, superior oblique paresis)
Pneumonia (e.g. upper lobe pneumonia)	Klippel–Feil syndrome
Cervical lymphadenitis	Dystonia
Muscular torticollis (sternomastoid tumour, CP)	Vertebral anomalies
Congenital abnormalities of cervical spine	Rheumatoid arthritis
	Hysteria
	Polymyalgia rheumatica
	Arnold–Chiari malformation

Misdiagnosis is due to:

1st mistake: failing to recognise subtle, non-specific presentation of meningitis.

2nd mistake: failing to differentiate the main other causes of neck stiffness.

1. Non-Specific Symptoms of Meningitis

- Neck stiffness due to meningitis is a straightforward diagnosis when presentation occurs with fever, headache, vomiting and neck stiffness in an ill-looking child. However, in infants including neonates, early presentations of meningitis are usually subtle and non-specific, with irritability, lethargy, body temperature instability, poor feeding, respiratory distress, shock with hypotension and seizures. Neck stiffness is commonly absent. Bulging fontanelle is a late sign.

- In older children, the classical signs of meningitis may not be apparent but rather with virus-like illness and a mixture of leg pain, drowsiness, confusion, neck pain, seizure and behavioural changes. Within few hours it can rapidly progress to septic shock, hypotension, DIC (disseminated intravascular coagulopathy) and death. Vigilance and high index of suspicion are required.

- Skin of a child with meningism should be carefully searched for any rash or petechiae of meningococcal septicaemia.

2. Non-Meningitis Neck Stiffness

Pneumonia

Children with an upper lobe pneumonia may present with meningism. Even if pneumonia is diagnosed, LP (lumbar puncture) is required to exclude concomitant meningitis. Diagnosis of pneumonia is based on the following:

- Community acquired pneumonia is defined: fever, clinical signs (cough, dyspnoea, tachypnoea, grunting and nasal flaring and referred pain) and chest-x ray infiltrates in a previously well child. Lower lobe pneumonia may cause lower abdominal pain mimicking acute appendicitis. Upper lobe pneumonia may cause meningism (increased CSF pressure, but CSF is otherwise normal).

- Findings include inspiratory crepitations and bronchial breathing on auscultation. Tachypnoea (>40/min aged >1 year, >50/min aged 2–12 months and >60/min aged <2 month) is the WHO defined criterion to diagnose pneumonia.

  - Wheezing, cough and fever may occur with mycoplasma infection.
  - Chest X-ray is diagnostic but it is often of limited value in distinguishing bacterial and viral. The presence of effusion and/or lobar consolidation suggests bacterial aetiology.
  - Isolation of the pathogens causing pneumonia is usually not possible in practice. Bacterial culture from the pharyngeal area or expectorated sputum is unreliable.

Torticollis
- Torticollis (wry neck) is characterised by tilting and rotation of the head to one side with the chin pointing in the opposite side. In infants, it is usually caused by shortening sternomastoid muscle following swelling formation (called sternomastoid tumour), or cranio-cervical vertebral abnormalities.
- Acquired ocular torticollis is caused by, e.g. strabismus or 6th cranial nerve palsy leading to torticollis as the child adopts a compensatory head position to regain binocular single vision. Non-ocular torticollis may be due to musculoskeletal trauma or posterior fossa tumour. Common result of either types of torticollis is facial asymmetry.
- Ocular torticollis is diagnosed by returning the head to normal position upon closing the affected eye, whereas torticollis due non-ocular causes persists during sleep or when the affected eye closes.

Dystonia
- Dystonia is a movement disorder characterised by intermittent or sustained muscle contracture causing abnormal posture. Causes of dystonia include inherited, degenerative or neoplastic diseases, or caused by drugs/toxins.
- There are no diagnostic criteria and the diagnosis is clinical by patterned twisting often initiated or worsened by voluntary action.

Acute Disseminated Encephalomyelitis (ADE)
- ADE compromises a group of inflammatory demyelinating diseases (e.g. multiple sclerosis) which manifests with fever, drowsiness, headache and vomiting, and most importantly, optic neuritis. Symptoms often follow 1-2 weeks after a viral infection.
- Presenting features are dominated by acute encephalopathy with multifocal neurological signs and fever.
- Diagnosis is established by certain criteria on MRI which include widespread demyelinating lesions located in the brain and spinal cord. CSF often shows mild lymphocytic pleocytosis with increased protein.

Further Reading

Mohseni S, Shojaiefard A, Khorgami Z, et al. Peripheral lymphadenopathy: approach and diagnostic tools. Iran J Med Sci. 2014;39(2 Suppl):158–70.

Muirhead S. Diagnostic approach to goitre in children. Paediatr Child Health. 2001;6(4):195–9.

Chapter 6
The Abdomen

6.1 Acute Abdominal Pain (AAP)

Introduction/Core Messages

- Abdominal pain is classified as visceral that is typically vague, dull, poorly localised, more likely aching. The pain usually originates from the internal organs in response to ischaemia, inflammation and/or distension. Visceral pain originating from the lower oesophagus, stomach is typically felt in the lower abdomen. Examples are inflammatory bowel disease or dyspepsia. Somatic pain is typically sharp, intense and well localised. Example of this type of pain is musculoskeletal injury such as arthritis. Referred pain is felt in distant areas of the same cutaneous dermatome as the affected organs, e.g. pneumonia or pharyngitis causing abdominal pain.

- The term "acute abdomen" refers to intra-abdominal condition, which usually requires a surgical intervention, such as appendicitis. This accounts to around 1% of all children presenting with AAP.

© Springer Nature Switzerland AG 2021   97
A. S. El-Radhi, *Avoiding Misdiagnosis in Pediatric Practice*,
In Clinical Practice, https://doi.org/10.1007/978-3-030-41750-5_6

- Bilious vomiting must always be taken seriously because of possible malrotation or volvulus.
- A young child with a mild abdominal pain, vomiting and with clinical signs of dehydration, but no ketones in the urine should be investigated to rule out an inborn error of metabolism.
- The main objective in dealing with AAP is to differentiate between benign and self-limited conditions, such as constipation or gastroenteritis, and more life-threatening surgical conditions such as volvulus or appendicitis. Without clear diagnostic criteria of the AP causes, unnecessary tests and wrong treatment are offered leading to more worries.

Differential Diagnosis

Common	Rare
Infantile colic	Crohn's disease
Gastroenteritis (GE)	Incarcerated hernia
Functional AP	Intestinal obstruction (e.g. Intussusception)
Constipation	Meckel's diverticulum
Appendicitis	Renal/gall bladder stones
Mesenteric adenitis (MA)	Hepatobiliary (e.g. pancreatitis, hepatitis)
Extra-intestinal (tonsillitis, UTI)	Henoch-Schönlein purpura
Exercise-related AP	Sickle cell anaemia

Misdiagnosis is due to:

1st mistake: not having or remembering basic knowledge when a child presents with acute AP.

2nd mistake: not considering extra-abdominal sources of AP (referred pain) in the differential diagnosis

3rd mistake: failing to recognise important non-surgical causes of acute AP.

4th mistake: little knowledge about exercise-related AP in the differential diagnosis.

5th mistake: failing to diagnose and differentiate surgical causes of acute AP.

1. Basic Knowledge of Acute AP

- Abdominal examination should be performed with extreme gentleness and compassion; careful hands-off inspection being the first step, followed by non-intimidating position of sitting down or kneeling to be at the same level with the child. A young child is best examined in parent's arms or lap. Distracting the child while palpating the abdomen is very helpful.
- It is worth asking the child to point with his/her finger to the area "where it hurts most".
- The closer the pain to the umbilicus, the less likely it is to be of organic disease.
- A student or a postgraduate doctor in an examination who hurts the child while examining the abdomen should expect a failure mark as a result.

  Clinical differentiation between non-surgical from surgical causes of AP may be difficult. Localisation of pain limited to one area of the abdomen helps clinicians identify the source of AP from the history in 80–90% of cases. Figure 6.1 shows the regions of the abdomen where the pain is usually localised. In general, pain localisation in one area of the abdomen is likely to be a sign of a disease in the underlying organ (Table 6.1). However, in children, particularly in young children, localisation of the pain is often difficult as the pain may originate from other areas of the body, e.g. lungs or genitalia. Therefore a comprehensive physical examination is necessary to establish a diagnosis.

2. Referred Abdominal Pain

  Referred pain is a pain perceived distant from its source. AP caused by referred pain is usually mild to moderate in severity and diffuse. Tenderness and rebound phenomenon are usually absent. When examining a child with AP, it is important not to confine the attention to the abdomen alone, but to do a comprehensive physical examination. Clinicians have to be aware of these distant sites and examining them if a diagnosis after initial abdominal examina-

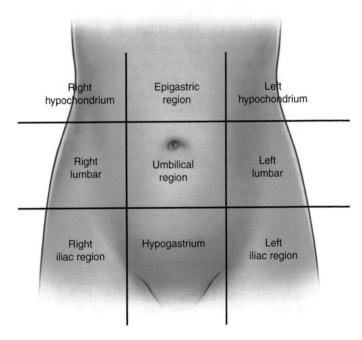

FIGURE 6.1

TABLE 6.1 Differential diagnosis of AAP according to pain localisation

Area	Diseases
Epigastric	Gastric: gastritis, peptic ulcer, pancreatitis, Biliary: cholangitis, cholecystitis
Right upper quadrant	Hepatitis, pulmonary: pneumonia
Right lower quadrant	Appendicitis
Left upper quadrant	Gastric: peptic ulcer, Renal: UTI, Pancreas: pancreatitis
Left lower quadrant	Irritable bowel syndrome (IBS)
Peri-umbilical	Functional (mostly psychogenic): non-organic, early appendicitis, colonic

tion could not be established. Examples of these extra-abdominal sites are:

- Groin pain caused by renal stones.
- Upper abdominal and shoulder pain caused by gall bladder infection or stones.
- Upper abdominal pain caused by pneumonia subsequent to diaphragmatic irritation.
- Upper respiratory tract infections, e.g. tonsillitis may produce upper or central AP.
- Testicular disease, spine or hip synovitis that can produce abdominal pain mimicking abdominal emergencies, e.g. appendicitis.

3. Non-surgical Causes of AAP
   Gastroenteritis

- The pain is usually crampy. Typical abdomen is non-distended, soft and mildly tender, with mild tenderness and little or no guarding. Diffuse abdominal pain occurs before diarrhoea begins.
- Vomiting usually precedes the diarrhoea by as much as 12–24 h.
- Associated diarrhoea is usually watery if the small intestine is involved (e.g. rotavirus enteritis) and bloody with mucus if the colon is involved (e.g. Shigella enteritis).

Mesenteric Adenitis (MA)
As mesenteric lymphnodes are usually localised in the right lower quadrant of abdomen. MA often mimic appendicitis. Distinguishing features include the following:

- History of an upper respiratory tract infection (URTI).
- Vomiting precedes the abdominal pain.
- Diffuse AP which is important sign to compare with localised AP of appendicitis.
- MA is a diagnosis of exclusion other causes, particularly appendicitis.
- Ultrasound scan or CT image may show enlarged mesenteric lymphnodes (5–15 mm), with thickened wall of the terminal ileum. Blood leukocytes and CRP are usu-

ally normal. Stool culture for the bacteria Yersinia should be performed.

Functional AP (Psychogenic AP)

- Affects usually older children and adolescents with a history of recurrent AP.
- AP is characterised by diffuse abdominal pain and mild tenderness.
- Associated psychological problems can often be elicited.
- Diagnosis should only be considered by excluding other causes of AP.

Urinary Tract Infection

- Presentation of UTI depends on the age of the child: Neonates with UTI usually present with symptoms and signs of sepsis. Infants and young children usually present with high fever (without a focus of infection), rigor, and vomiting. Older children present with loan and suprapubic pain and tenderness. Other typical symptoms in older children (usually girls) are dysuria, frequency and urgency of urination, and secondary enuresis.
- Diagnosis is established by urinalysis and culture.

Constipation

- Constipation involves fewer than 3 stools per week with faecal incontinence, large stools, palpable impacted stool masses in the rectum, posturing and painful defecation.
- Constipation causing abdominal pain is commonly reported. Constipation should not be accepted as the cause of abdominal pain without consideration of alternative diagnoses.
- If constipation is causing abdominal pain, it is usually mild, diffuse or absent.

Crohn's Disease (CD)

- CD is a chronic inflammatory disease that affects the gastrointestinal tract from the mouth to the anus.
- Children usually present with **fever**, diarrhoea, anorexia, oral ulcers, perianal skin tag/fistula, growth failure, vague crampy abdominal pain, often mimicking appendicitis and weight loss. Extra-intestinal features include arthropathy, scleritis and erythema nodosum.
- High CRP, anaemia and thrombocytosis are fairly characteristic.
- Diagnosis is by colonoscopy with biopsy, barium meal, MRI or CT scan.
- Stool calprotectin can differentiate between IBD (Inflammatory bowel diseases) and IBS (Irritable bowel syndrome).

Pancreatitis

- Risk factors are intake of the anticonvulsant valproate, hyperlipidaemia, biliary tract disorder or family history of pancreatitis.
- Abdominal pain/tenderness, which is persistent, radiating to the back.
- Vomiting/retching (incidence about 75%).
- Fever/chills (incidence in about 25%).
- Elevated serum lipase and amylase level ($>3\times$ times the upper limit of normal).
- Imaging studies: ultrasonography and CT scan.

4. Exercise-Related AP

- This is a common transient complaint following exercise, and referred to as "stitch".
- It is mostly localised in the right mid abdomen along the subcostal border, sharp or stabbing occurring particularly after running and horse riding.
- Often the pain is referring to the shoulder which is the referred site from tissue innervated by phrenic nerve.
- Food or drinks (particularly hypertonic beverages) prior to the exercise is a risk factor predisposing to this type of AP.
- The pain is often relieved by deep breathing.

5. Surgical Conditions Presenting with AP

AP due to acute surgical conditions is usually sudden in onset, severe, progressive and colicky with localised tenderness. Pain generally precedes vomiting, while the reverse is true with medical cases. Children with midline pain without worsening pain or vomiting, with mild or moderate pain tend to have nonspecific benign AP.

Summary of diagnostic features of the two groups, surgical and non-surgical causes, with AP is shown in Table 6.2:

Diagnostic features of the most common surgical conditions are:

Appendicitis

- Initial vague, crampy abdominal pain, poorly localised in the peri-umbilical area followed by nausea.
- Within 6–48 h, the pain migrates to right lower quadrant followed by vomiting and fever.
- Fever, ranges 38–39 °C, is present in 80%.
- Right lower quadrant tenderness with rebound phenomenon on examination.
- Pain worsens with coughing, percussion, hopping.
- Young children with appendicitis often present with acute abdomen due to perforation. These children typically have longer history of pain, greater systemic effect, high fever, more generalized tenderness and absent bowel sounds.
- Abnormal laboratory findings: leukocytosis and high CRP. Ultrasound scan can differentiate conditions mimicking appendicitis and suggest the diagnosis. CT scan is a very important image technique when ultrasonography fails to give a definite diagnosis: It can confirm an enlarged appendix (> 7mm transverse diameter and significant wall enhancement).

Volvulus

- Volvulus involves twisting of the bowel around a fixed point. Typical age is 2 months to 2 years.

TABLE 6.2 Distinguishing features between surgical and non-surgical causes of AP

Surgical	Non-surgical
History	
• Acute, severe pain, increasing in intensity	Midline or generalised, intensity stable
• Pain precedes vomiting	Long or recurrent pain episodes
• Bilious vomiting	Vomiting absent or precedes pain onset
• Haematochezia (rectal bleeding)	
Physical examination	
• Ill appearing, lethargic	Non-ill appearing
• Abdominal distension	Abdomen non-distended
• Localised, rebound tenderness	Diffuse tenderness
• Rigidity, guarding	No rigidity, or rebound tenderness
• Absent or high-pitches bowel sounds	Normal bowel sounds

- Newborns present with acute symptoms of bilious vomiting, abdominal distension and other symptoms and signs of intestinal obstruction. Toddlers and older children may present with recurrent AP.
- Ultrasound scan examination is diagnostic.

Intussusception
- This is one of the most common causes of acute abdomen affecting particularly children aged 6 month-2 years.
- Onset is characterised by initial vomiting with absence of stool passage, followed by paroxysms (every 10–20 min) of colicky AP. The child is in distress, crying and

ill-looking, but well between these paroxysms. There is usually a palpable mass and a bloody red, currant-jelly stools or haematochezia.

- Reduction by air or barium enema under ultrasound guidance is diagnostic and therapeutic.

Incarcerated Hernia

- Incarcerated hernia is the most common and serious complication of inguinal hernia. Around 15% of the childhood hernias become incarcerated.
- Children present with sudden crying and visible mass in the groin or scrotum or in the major labia.
- Physical examination reveals local irreducible mass with obvious tenderness.
- If the incarceration time is <12 h, manual reduction can be tried which confirms the diagnosis.
- Ultrasound scan is diagnostic.

6.2   Recurrent Abdominal Pain (RAP)

Introduction/Core Messages
- RAP is significant because it is responsible for high rate of morbidity, missed school days, high use of health resources and parental anxiety. It is defined as "at least 3 recurrent episodes of pain, severe enough to affect child's activities, over a period of at least 3 months, and the symptoms cannot be attributed to another medical condition.
- RAP is characterised by symptoms-free interval, healthy appearance of the child and absence of abnormalities on examination. Organic diseases tend to have progressive course and presence of abnormalities on examination.

- Recently (Rome criteria), the term of functional gastrointestinal disorders (FGIDs) was introduced that includes irritable bowel syndrome (IBS), functional dyspepsia (epigastric pain, postprandial distress, early satiation), and functional abdominal pain.
- Parasites, such as giardia, are common and important cause of RAP in developing countries.

Differential Diagnosis

Common	Rare
Infantile colic (evening colic)	Child abuse
Gastro-oesophageal reflux	Coeliac disease
Food allergy/intolerance	Inflammatory bowel diseases (Crohn's disease, ulcerative colitis)
Functional AP disorders (FAPD)	Stones in the urinary tract and gall bladder
Functional dyspepsia	Meckel's diverticulum
Irritable bowel syndrome	Familial Mediterranean fever
Abdominal migraine	Parasites (e.g. Giardia)
Functional AP (FAP)	Sickle cell anaemia
	Recurrent UTI

Misdiagnosis is due to:

1st mistake: failing to differentiate organic from non-organic causes of RAP.

2nd mistake: failing to differentiate the most common causes of RAP in infancy.

3rd mistake: failing to differentiate common causes of RAP in older children.

4th mistake: not considering rare causes of RAP (e.g. child abuse).

1. Differentiating Organic from Non-Organic RAP
   In Favour of Non-organic RAB:

   - The vast majority of cases with RAP have a non-organic aetiology.
   - AP is central peri-umbilical and does not radiate elsewhere.
   - Absence of abnormality on physical examination, without guarding, rebound and rigidity, and normal investigation.
   - Absence of alarm symptoms (see below).

   In Favour of Organic RAP

   - Abdominal pain is localised away from the umbilicus, and/or radiating elsewhere.
   - Young children < 4 years of age, weight loss, falling off growth centile, persistent pain in the right or left upper or right lower quadrant of the abdomen or in the supra-pubic area, or association with significant vomiting, persistent diarrhoea or unexplained fever.
   - Other alarm features include family history of inflammatory bowel diseases, pain associated with night-waking, oral and/or perianal lesions, arthritis or hepatomegaly that suggest non-functional causes of abdominal pain.

2. Causes of RAP in Infancy
   Infantile Colic (see also Chapter of General Systemic).

   - Recurrent crying episodes in an infant who draws the legs up and appears to be in pain are considered colic.
   - Infant colic is defined as irritability paroxysms with fussiness or crying that starts and ends without clear reasons, lasting at least 3 h/day, 3 days/week, for at least 3 weeks in a healthy baby.
   - It usually begins aged 2 weeks and significantly improves by the age of 3–4 months. Characteristically, the attack begins suddenly, is continuous, with flushed face, tense

abdomen, fisted hands and drawing up of legs. Around 5% of cases have organic causes. Crying may be a baby's way of communication. As children grow older, they find different ways to communicate.

- Colic typically is noted more in the afternoon and evening (commonly 6–10 p.m.) suggesting that events at home (e.g. mum is busy with households; child being left alone) could be the major cause. This evening colic used to be the most common diagnosis of infantile colic; this is being replaced by GO-reflux.
- Persistent crying beyond four months of age has been associated with long-term psychological and behavioural problems, including hyperactivity and migraine.

Gastroesophageal Reflux (GOR)

- GOR is common in infants, and refers to as the involuntary retrograde passage of gastric contents into the oesophagus with or without regurgitation and/or vomiting. The vast majority of infants with GOR do well aged 6–12 months.
- Clinical manifestations are either general (discomfort, irritability, feeding refusal, and dystonic neck posturing = Sandifer syndrome), or gastrointestinal (epigastric pain, dysphagia, haematemesis and regurgitation). Regurgitation is the most frequent symptoms and is present in almost all children with GOR. Red flag symptoms and signs include weight loss, lethargy, excessive irritability, presence of fever, and onset of regurgitation/vomiting > 6 months and their persistence > 12–18 months of age. Complications of GOR include peptic oesophagitis, gastrointestinal bleeding, laryngitis and recurrent aspiration pneumonia.
- Investigations include barium contrast, ultrasonography, endoscopy, oesophageal pH-monitoring, multichannel intraluminal oesophageal electrical impedance.
- Pyloric stenosis is differentiated from GO-reflux by projectile vomiting in the first 2–3 weeks of life in a baby who is hungry with visible gastric peristalsis and a palpation of an "olive" in the right upper quadrant. With reflux, children vomit during or immediately after feeding.

Cow's Milk Protein Allergy (CMPA)

- Immediate reaction of CMPA (IgE-mediated) occurs within 2 hours of milk intake and manifests as gastrointestinal (GI) (vomiting, diarrhoea, abdominal pain), skin (urticaria) respiratory symptoms (wheezy).
- Non-IgE mediated CMPA is characterised by delayed onset (two hours to several days), with symptoms confined to the GI-tract (colic, GOR, diarrhoea, enterocolitis, and blood and/or mucus in stools), and skin (pruritis, erythema, and atopic eczema).
- Investigation for IgE mediated CMPA includes skin prick test (SPT) and specific serum IgE tests. There are no validated tests to confirm non-IgE mediated CMPA. Elimination of cow's milk and dairy products for two weeks and replacing the milk by extensively hydrolysed formula will help establish the diagnosis.

Lactose Intolerance (LI)

- Cow's milk contains about 5g lactose per 100 ml. Yoghurt contains about 50% of that, and cheese has low lactose content.
- LI is defined as the onset of abdominal symptoms following lactose ingestion. It usually occurs secondary to viral (e.g. rotavirus) gastroenteritis causing lactase deficiency and thus an inability to split the disaccharide lactose into galactose and glucose.
- Lactose malabsorption (LM) is passage of lactose into large intestine as a consequence of lactase deficiency. LM is a precondition for LI, and only some individuals with LM are lactose intolerant.
- Typical symptoms include abdominal pain, bloating, diarrhoea and malabsorption.
- Diagnosis is established by low faecal pH (< 5.3), positive reducing substances in stool, and positive hydrogen breath test ($H_2 >20$ ppm over baseline indicates LM). A lactose challenge test (12.5–25 g lactose) is also available.

3. Causes of RAP in Older Children

Functional Dyspepsia (FD)

FD includes one or more of the following bothersome symptoms of at least 4 days/month for at least 2 months:

- Postprandial fullness
- Early satiation
- Epigastric pain or burning
- Symptoms cannot be fully explained by another medical condition

Irritable Bowel Syndrome (IBS)

The prevalence of IBS in the population is high (11%), and females are more affected than males. Diagnostic criteria are abdominal pain or discomfort occurring at least 4 days per month associated with one or more of the following:

- Associated stool irregularity (constipation-predominately, diarrhoea-predominately or mixed). With constipation, the pain does not resolve after defecation; if it does it is functional constipation but not IBS.
- Associated comorbidities include overactive bladder, migraine and psychiatric problems (e.g. anxiety).
- Symptoms cannot be fully explained by another medical condition.
- Clinical presentation of inflammatory bowel diseases (IBD) often overlaps with IBS. Stool calprotectin has proved to be very useful in the differential diagnosis between IBD and IBS: low calprotectin ($< 50\mu g/g$) makes IBD unlikely.

Abdominal Migraine

- Paroxysmal episodes of moderate to severe localized peri-umbilical, or diffuse abdominal lasting at least an hour. Pain is severe enough to interfere with daily normal activities.
- Accompanied features include pallor, nausea, vomiting, anorexia, headache and photophobia.
- Episodes are separated by weeks to months symptom-free intervals.
- Common family history of migraine.

- Symptoms cannot be attributed to another medical condition.

Functional Abdominal Pain (FAP)

- Although the term of recurrent AP is frequently used, the current preference is to use functional AP, which is defined by at least 3 bouts of pain severe enough to affect activities over a period of at least 3 months. The AP occurs in the absence of anatomical abnormalities, inflammation or tissue damage.
- The diagnosis is clinical with a normal physical findings and no alarming symptoms and signs.
- Although the cornerstone of the diagnosis is an accurate history, few selected tests such as urinalysis can be performed before the final diagnosis of FAP is made.

Crohn's Disease (See Section of Acute AP)

Constipation (see also Next Section)

- Pain in constipation is often overrated as a diagnostic entity.
- The diagnosis of constipation should not be made because no other cause except constipation is elicited from the history and examination.

Food Allergy/Intolerance

- Food allergy is adverse reactions to a specific food antigen mediated by immunological process in a susceptible individual. Food intolerance is non-immunological reactions mediated by toxin, drug, or enzyme deficiency. Typically, food allergy/intolerance begins in the first two years of life.
- Symptoms usually involve the skin, gut, and respiratory systems. While allergic reaction to milk and egg usually disappears with age, allergy to nuts and seafood persist.
- Food allergy/intolerance is among the most common causes of RAP in an otherwise healthy child. Eliminating the suspected food item (particularly milk or wheat) for

about two weeks is the best diagnostic and therapeutic tool. Blood or skin testing is only useful in IgE-mediated reactions.

4. Rare Causes of RAP
   Child Abuse

- Children who have been abused (physical, neglect, sexual) display a variety of symptoms including RAP. Associated features that can lead to the diagnosis of abuse include sleep disturbance, night terrors, changes of behaviour and personality, unexplained skin bruises, inflicted cigarette burns, retinal haemorrhages and intra-oral injury.
- Diagnosis is usually based on a discrepancy between the history and the clinical findings.
- Radiological skeletal survey may be indicated.

Parasites (e.g. Giardia lamblia, Cryptosporidium Species).

- Parasitic infections involving the GI-tract manifest as RAP, bloating, diarrhoea, and abdominal distension. Giardia is classically associated with foul-smelling watery diarrhoea.
- In children presenting with severe symptoms due to parasitic infection, immune deficiency should be considered.
- Stool for parasites should be considered in any child with intestinal symptoms following visit abroad.

Familial Mediterranean Fever (FMF)
Diagnostic Criteria of FMF are:

- Recurring episodes of fever at irregular intervals over a course of many months.
- Pain in the abdomen (peritonitis), the chest (pleuritis) or the joints (arthritis). A prodromal period of 4–12 h is usually present and is characterized by loss of appetite and abdominal pain due to peritonitis. About 6–10 h later, fever (38.5 °C to as high as 40 °C) occurs and rapid recovery ensues within 24–72 h. Many patients

undergo at least one abdominal operation for suspected appendicitis before FMF is diagnosed. Recurrent oral aphthae are often present. Pericarditis occurs in less than 1%. Amyloidosis is the principal long-term complication of FMF.
- Genetic testing (MEFV mutation) confirms the diagnosis.

6.3   Abdominal Distension

Introduction/Core Messages
- Abdominal distension is defined as an increase of girth of the abdomen caused by air, fluid, stool, mass or organomegaly. It is a common clinical finding that must be evaluated carefully.
- History is of paramount importance in giving a diagnostic clue, e.g. duration of the distension (acute or chronic), any weight loss, diarrhoea or vomiting and is the vomiting bile-stained?

Differential Diagnosis

Common	Rare
Physiological in toddlers	Storage diseases (Glycogen storage)
Malabsorption (Coeliac disease, Giardia)	Hirschsprung's diseases
Intestinal obstruction	Ascites (e.g. nephrotic syndrome, SLE)
Constipation	Ovarian cyst
Abdominal mass (tumour, hepatosplenomegaly)	Polycystic renal disease
Aerophagia (functional or pathological)	Hydatid cyst (in the tropics)

Misdiagnosis is due to:

1st mistake: failing to recognise physiological causes of abdominal distension.

2nd mistake: failing to differentiate pathological causes of abdominal distension.

1. Physiological Abdominal Distension

- In children, 70% of the bowel gas comes from swallowed air. Air swallowing is physiological in newborns and infants.
- Many toddlers, who are thriving and well, often have a mild and harmless abdominal distension. This condition may be associated with toddler's diarrhoea.
- Aerophagia: Physiological functional aerophagia refers to air swallowing without significant gastrointestinal symptoms. Typical presentation: no abdominal distension in the morning followed by progressive abdominal distension during the day.

2. Pathological Abdominal Distension
   Pathological Aerophagia

- Pathological aerophagia is caused by excessive and inappropriate swallowing of air, and is associated with abdominal distension and pain, belching, burping and repetitive flatulence that lasts >12 weeks/year. As with physiological aerophagia, no abdominal distension occurs in the morning followed by progressive abdominal distension during the day. Audible swallowing sounds are pathognomonic of this condition.
- Pathological aerophagia commonly occurs in the flowing situations:

  - Disabled children who are frequently unable to burp. Associated constipation often limits the elimination of flatus.
  - Children with irritable bowel syndrome (IBS), commonly associated with bloating.
  - Severe constipation causing more abdominal distension than bloating.
  - Tracheo-oesophageal fistula.

Malabsorption

- Malabsorption is failure of absorption of nutrients resulting from luminal/mucosal mal-digestion and/or inadequate mucosal absorption. Clinically it manifests as diarrhoea, steatorrhoea, (with pale-greasy and bulky stools) malnutrition, weight loss, abdominal pain and anaemia. These features usually result from carbohydrate and fat malabsorption only.
- Coeliac disease (chronic small-intestinal, autoimmune enteropathy precipitated by exposure to dietary gluten) is diagnosed on clinical features of malabsorption and serological markers of CD including endomysial, and anti-tissue transglutaminase (anti-tTG)-IgA.
- Physical examination alone is insufficient in establishing a specific diagnosis for malabsorption. Although stools in steatorrhoea have a characteristic appearance, the diagnosis can be confirmed by Sudan stain which tests for the number of fat globules (> 20/hpf is abnormal). Pancreatic insufficiency can be screened by measuring faecal elastase-1. Once this diagnosis is suspected, sweat test to confirm or exclude cystic fibrosis is required. The diagnosis of carbohydrate malabsorption is suggestive by low stool pH (< 5.3), by positive reducing substances in stool (using clinitest), positive hydrogen breath test, and by using D-xylose test (normally > 20mg/dl) following an oral dose of D-xylose.

Constipation (See Next Section)

Intra-Abdominal Mass

- Abdominal masses include small-intestinal lymphoma, gastric teratoma and cysts. In the tropics protozoal and helminthic infections are common.
- Diagnosis is established by imaging with ultrasound and MRI.

Intestinal Obstruction

- Cardinal signs of congenital intestinal obstruction include maternal polyhydramnios, bilious vomiting, and failure to pass meconium in 24 h of life, in addition to abdominal distension. Intestinal atresia, Hirschsprung's disease, malrotation and meconium ileus (occurs in 15% of all cases cystic fibrosis cases) are the most common diseases. Acquired intestinal obstruction includes intussusception and incarcerated hernia.

- Distal intestinal obstruction (e.g. caused by Hirschsprung's disease) manifests with early abdominal distension and late vomiting, while proximal intestinal (e.g. caused by duodenal atresia) manifests with early vomiting and no abdominal distension. Bilious vomiting and/or intestinal fluid levels suggest intestinal obstruction.
- Bilious vomiting must be taken seriously because of the possibility of malrotation with volvulus.

Tropics

- Causes of abdominal distension in the tropics differ from those in developed countries. Parasites (e.g. Giardia, Cryptosporidium) are common causing in addition to diarrhoea, abdominal distension and weight loss.
- Microscopical or ELISA antigen identification of faecal Giardia and Cryptosporidium cysts.

6.4   Constipation

Introduction/Core Messages
- Infrequent defecation is common in breast-fed babies who may not have a stool for 10 days. There should be no intervention as long as babies are thriving, feeding well, have no abdominal distension and pass stools without pain or blood.
- In older children, the most common reason of constipation is withholding stool for fear of having a bowel movement following an experience of a painful defecation.
- Faecal incontinence is a common complication of constipation occurring in about 80% of cases. It is defined as voluntary or involuntary passage of faeces into the underwear or in socially inappropriate

places, in a child with a developmental age of at least 4 years.
- Faecal incontinence not related to constipation (non-retentive), and organic causes (e.g. anorectal malformation) are comparatively uncommon.

Differential Diagnosis

Common	Rare
Common functional constipation	
Normal variants of breast-fed	Hypothyroidism
Associated neurodisability	Hypercalcaemia
Irritable bowel syndrome	Intestinal obstruction
Drugs	Increased output (polyuria, vomiting) Coeliac disease

Misdiagnosis is due to:

1st mistake: failing to define constipation.

2nd mistake: failing to differentiate functional causes of constipation.

3rd mistake: failing to distinguish organic causes of constipation.

1. Defining Functional Constipation
   - Rome IV diagnostic criteria for functional constipation at developmental age of >4 years require at least 2 of the following symptoms: Two or fewer defections in the toilet/week, at least one episode of faecal incontinence/week.
   - In addition to a history of retentive posturing, history of painful defecation, hard stool, large faecal mass in the rectum and stools that may obstruct the toilet.

2. Causes of Functional Constipation
   - By far the most common cause of constipation is functional, accounting or 90-95% of all cases. Organic causes (see next section) are rare in practice (around 5%).

- Pain in passing hard stools in early childhood is the principal factor for childhood constipation.
- Risk factors for constipation include poor dietary habit, obesity, milk intolerance/allergy and maltreatment that leads to stress with alteration of gastrointestinal motility.
- Faecal incontinence is usually due to "overflow" to faecal retention (in >80% of cases). Other causes are behavioural/emotional.
- Parents may interpret withholding stool as pushing, and faecal incontinence as diarrhoea. Explanation should be provided for both phenomena.

3. Causes of Non-Functional Organic Constipation

- Red flags for possible existence of organic constipation include delayed of meconium beyond 48 hours of life, bilious vomiting, abdominal distension and associated failure to thrive.
- Hirschsprung's disease is the commonest cause of neonatal intestinal obstruction; 80% are male. It is caused by an absence of enteric ganglia in the submucosal and mesenteric plexuses. Down's syndrome is the most common associated genetic disorder. The diagnosis is based on a combination of:

  - Clinical features: delayed passage of meconium, meconium ileus, bilious vomiting and abdominal distension. The rectum is usually empty on examination. Older children present with variable degrees of distended abdomen and infrequent defection.
  - A plain abdominal x-ray may show dilated segment proximal to the obstructed bowel segment. The diagnosis is confirmed by rectal biopsy showing aganglionosis along with high content of acetyl cholinesterase. Calretinin immunohistochemistry has emerged as an important diagnostic tool.

- Other non-functional causes of constipation include hypercalcaemia (see Section of Blood in Urine), ectopic anus, hypothyroidism and congenital megacolon.

6.5   Diarrhoea

Introduction/Core Messages

- Most diarrhoeal diseases in children living in developed countries are viral (75–90% of cases), mild and self-limited, and do not require hospitalization or laboratory evaluation. Diarrhoea is usually watery, large and non-bloody. In developing countries, diarrhoea is often severe with high rate of deaths. Frequent, small bloody stools with mucus suggest colitis.

- Large watery diarrhoea in association with diffuse abdominal pain and vomiting is typical for enteritis (usually termed gastroenteritis), whereas small frequent, bloody stools and lower abdominal pain are very suggestive of colitis.

- In children with vomiting alone, alternative diagnoses rather than gastroenteritis should be considered.

- With widespread use of rotavirus vaccine beginning in 2006, a substantial decrease in disease prevalence, morbidity and mortality has been achieved.

- The most important aspect of evaluation of diarrhoeal case is to determine the level of dehydration. Concentrated urine (orange colour) suggests mild dehydration, infrequent and small amount of urine suggests moderate and anuria means severe dehydration. If a child is alert and playful, the degree of dehydration is insignificant.

- Laxative-induced diarrhoea (induced illness) is rare but should not be missed. The diarrhoea is usually chronic or recurrent. Carer of the child has often an underlying psychiatric disturbance.

Differential Diagnosis

Common	Rare
Acute infective enteritis, GE	Acrodermatitis enteropathica
Milk protein/lactose intolerance	Inflammatory bowel disease (IBD)
Antibiotic induced	Primary disaccharide deficiency
Post-infectious lactose/protein intolerance	Short bowel syndrome
Coeliac disease	Nosocomial diarrhoea
Toddler's diarrhoea	Pseudomembranous colitis (drug-induced)
Irritable bowel syndrome Malabsorption	Munchausen syndrome by proxy

Misdiagnosis is due to:

1st mistake: failing to define diarrhoea.

2nd mistake: failing to consider extra-intestinal causes of diarrhoea.

3rd mistake: failing to establish causes of persistent diarrhoea.

1. What is Diarrhoea?

- Diarrhoea is defined as the passage of 3 or more loose or liquid stools per 24 hours (or more frequent passage than is normal for the individual). Frequent accompanied symptoms include vomiting, fever, nausea and abdominal pain (AP). Acute diarrhoea lasts by definition < 2 weeks. Frequent passage of formed stools is not diarrhoea, nor is passing of loose, "pasty" stools by breast-fed babies.

- Toddler's "diarrhoea" (functional diarrhoea) is the most common cause of chronic "diarrhoea" without failure to thrive. Excessive fruit juice and fructose consumption may play a role in the pathophysiology of this condition.

- Toddler's diarrhoea is common and should not be misdiagnosed as GE. These children are healthy and thriving, passing 3–5 soft stools daily, often containing undigested food particles (e.g. carrots, peas). It is self-limiting and resolve spontaneously when at school age.

2. Extra-Intestinal Causes of Diarrhoea

- About 15-20% of diarrhoeal diseases are not caused by infection of the gastrointestinal tract, but are due to systemic or other organ infection. The infection may be UTI, sepsis, pneumonia, malaria, Lyme disease or appendicitis.
- The diagnosis is considered when the general condition of the child is too unwell to be explained by the usually mild diarrhoea. Stool culture are usually negative but the results of tests of the extra-intestinal disease, e.g. urine or blood culture are positive.

3. Persistent Diarrhoea (PD)

- Diarrhoea lasting for >2 weeks is termed persistent or protracted diarrhoea (chronic diarrhoea lasts 30 days or longer). PD leads to long-term morbidity due to malabsorption of key nutrients caused by blunting villi and submucosal inflammation. PD may be due to infection by:
  - Giardia lamblia or Cyclospora species,
  - Bacteria such as enterotoxigenic E. coli, and
  - Viruses such as adenoviruses and noroviruses.

- Complications of PD include monosaccharide (glucose, fructose, glucose-galactose), disaccharide (sucrose, lactose, maltose) malabsorption, congenital chloride diarrhoea (causing watery diarrhoea) and pancreatic insufficiency (causing fatty diarrhoea).
- Carbohydrate malabsorption causing watery diarrhoea is confirmed by temporary withdrawal of milk and dairy products (which is diagnostic and therapeutic), reduced stool pH of < 5.3, positive reducing substance > 0.5% in

stool and positive hydrogen breath test. Pancreatic insufficiency is confirmed by cessation of diarrhoea after enzyme replacement therapy.

6.6   Gastrointestinal Bleeding

Introduction/Core Messages

- Gastrointestinal bleeding (GIB) is a common condition, and can occur from the mouth to the anus.
- An upper GIB (oesophagus, stomach and duodenum) that originates proximal to the ligament of Treitz (at the duodenal-jejunal junction), leads to haematemesis, coffee-ground vomiting and black tarry stools (melena). An upper GIB is uncommon in children but potentially life-threatening condition.
- Lower GIB originating from areas below the ligament of Treitz (small bowel, colon) produces bright red blood that has not been into contact with gastric juice.
- Bright blood mixed with loose stools suggests bleeding site above the rectum (colitis, e.g. infectious or ulcerative colitis). Beyond the neonatal period, anal fissures are the most common cause of rectal bleeding. The child presents with painful defecation and small blood streaks on the surface of the stool.
- Important factors in the differential diagnosis of GI bleeding: age of the child, the presence of absence of anal pain during blood passage and the presence or absence of diarrhoea.
- Children who present with persistent or recurrent iron-deficiency anaemia, occult GIB should be excluded by checking the stool for blood.

Differential Diagnosis

Common	Rare
Neonatal (well baby)	Inflammatory bowel disease
Swallowed maternal blood	Peptic ulcer
Vitamin K deficiency	Intussusception
Neonatal (unwell baby)	Meckel's diverticulum
Disseminated intravascular	
coagulopathy	
Older children	Thrombocytopenia/volvulus
Anal fissure	Polyp
Thrombocytopenia	Haemorrhagic diseases
Cow's milk protein	Mallory–Weiss syndrome
Henoch–Schönlein purpura	Haemolytic uraemic syndrome
	Hereditary haemorrhagic
	telangiectasia
	Hookworm infections

Misdiagnosis is due to:

1st mistake: failing to recognise conditions mimicking rectal bleeding.

2nd mistake: failing to differentiate causes of neonatal bleeding.

3rd mistake: failing to differentiate common causes of rectal bleeding in older children.

1. Conditions that can be Mistaken as Rectal Bleeding

- Urate crystals may appear on baby's nappy during the first few days of life that can be mistaken as blood. It is usually associated with concentrated urine. Offering extra fluid to the baby should eliminate these crystals.
- Multiple food items (e.g. red or black licorice, blueberries, large amounts of beets, red gelatine) and medications (e.g. iron supplement, bismuth such as Pepto-Bismol tablets) can cause red or black stools.
- If a change in stool colour cannot be explained for a dietary or medication reason, blood in stool should be

excluded by absence of red blood cells microscopically and negative faecal occult blood.

2. Recognising Neonatal Bleeding

- It is worth noting that infants up to the age of 3–4 months have physiological prolongation of PTT, and that abnormal PT and PTT only occur when coagulation factor levels are 40%.
- Rectal bleeding in a healthy neonate is most often maternal in origin swallowed either during delivery or breast feeding. The Apt test is performed on gastric aspirate or stool to rule out the presence of maternal blood swallowed during delivery or from a bleeding breast. Laboratory tests are normal (Table 6.3).
- Protein-induced colitis may occur in cow's milk protein allergy, which is a benign inflammatory colitis resulting from non-IgE-mediated immune reaction to ingested cow's milk protein. Elimination of the milk results in normal stools. Eosinophilic infiltration of the recto-sigmoid mucosa is characteristic.

TABLE 6.3 Differential diagnosis of common causes of neonatal bleeding

	Platelets	PT	PTT	Likely diagnosis
Healthy	N	N	N	Swallowed maternal blood
	N	N	N	Protein-induced colitis
	↓	N	N	Immune thrombocytopenia
	N	↑	↑	Haemorrhagic disease of newborn
	N	N	↑	Hereditary clotting factors deficiencies
Unwell	↓	↑	↑	DIC
	↓	N	N	Platelets consumption (e.g. infection)
	N	↑	↑	Liver disease

PT prothrombin time, *PTT* partial thromboplastin time, *N* normal; ↓ = low; ↑ = prolonged

- Haemorrhagic disease of the newborn (HDN) usually occurs within 48 h of birth with gastrointestinal bleeding in infants who were not given vitamin K prophylaxis. The platelet count is normal; PT and PTT are prolonged.
- Immune thrombocytopenia may occur in infants of mothers with idiopathic thrombocytopenic purpura (ITP), or disseminated lupus erythematosus. Platelet count is low, and PT and PTT are normal.
- Hereditary clotting factors deficiencies (e.g. Von Willebrand disease, haemophilia) are associated with normal platelet count, normal PT and prolonged PTT. Bleeding time is prolonged.
- Disseminated intravascular coagulation (DIC) is usually caused by infection or hypoxia. The baby usually appears unwell with petechiae and gastrointestinal haemorrhage. The platelet count is low, and PT and PTT are prolonged. Serum fibrin split products are present and fragmented red blood cells are seen in blood smear.

3. Rectal Bleeding in Older Children

Important factors in the differential diagnosis of GI bleeding: age of the child, the presence of absence of anal pain during blood passage and the presence or absence of diarrhoea. The two possible sources of rectal bleeding are upper GI bleeding, usually causing melaena, and lower GI bleed producing bright red blood and caused by anorectal disorders such as fissures, distal polyps and haemorrhoids. However, massive upper GI bleeding can produce bright red blood per rectum if the GI transient time is rapid.

Endoscopy is the method of choice for evaluating GIB that should be performed within 24 h of presentation, after stabilization of the child. It has also therapeutic role for polyps and ulcers.

Anal Fissure

- Anal fissure is commonly associated with constipation and pain on defection. Blood streaks are seen on stool.

- Inspection of the anal area usually establishes the diagnosis.

Henoch–Schönlein Purpura=HSP (newly termed: IgA vasculitis).

- The abdominal pain in HSP may be severe and can lead to laparotomy, particularly if it precedes the skin rash and joint manifestations. Buttocks, arm and legs should be searched for urticarial lesions or petechiae.
- HSP is the most common vasculitis in children with IgA immune deposits affecting small blood vessels. Renal involvement occurs in 20–40% of cases, determining long-term prognosis.
- Distribution of the purpura can offer important clues to the diagnosis: the lesions are predominately on the shins, feet and buttocks; in ITP, there is bruising and bleeding from the gums and mucous membrane.
- Specific diagnostic tests are absent. Urine should repeatedly be tested for proteinuria and haematuria.

Polyps

- Juvenile colonic polyp (inflammatory polyp) is the most common GI tumour in childhood affecting 3–4%. Most common age at presentation is 2–8 years.
- Painless rectal bleeding with normal stool pattern is suggestive of the presence of juvenile polyp.

Meckel's Diverticulum

- Meckel's diverticulum should strongly be suspected at any age if bleeding is massive and accompanied by both bright and dark red stools. Other symptoms include abdominal pain (related to gastric or pancreatic ectopic tissues) and intestinal obstruction. An inflamed Meckel's may be mistaken for an appendicitis.
- Investigation includes abdominal X-ray, ultrasound scan, CT-scan and MRI (all have low specificity and sensitivity). Diagnosis can be established by nuclear scans with Tc-99 that can visualize the diverticulum.

Inflammatory Bowel Diseases

- GI bleeding is less common with Crohn's disease than with ulcerative colitis (UC). The former presents with the triad of anaemia, loss of weight and abdominal pain. UC manifests with bloody and mucus diarrhoea, urgency and tenesmus.
- Diagnostic radiology includes endoscopy with biopsy. Stool culture should be performed to exclude infective enteritis.

6.7   Jaundice

Introduction/Core Messages

- Jaundice is very common during the neonatal period: 60% of term and 80% of preterm babies become jaundiced with indirect hyperbilirubinaemia (IHB) in the first few days of life, mainly due to breakdown of red blood cells.
- Indirect bilirubin is fat-soluble and can cause brain damage and kernicterus. After the neonatal period, infection remains the most common cause of jaundice worldwide.
- Direct bilirubin is more serious than indirect one as it is associated with hepatocellular damage and cholestasis that can lead to bleeding tendency and liver cirrhosis.
- Hepatitis A (HA) used to be a common infection, but its incidence rate has declined significantly in developed countries.
- Liver function tests should include total bilirubin and direct bilirubin (for persistent jaundice >2w), alkaline phosphatase, prothrombin time (PT), partial thromboplastin time (PTT), albumin, blood group and Rh-status of the mother and infant, and Coombs test.

Differential Diagnosis

Common	Rare
Indirect hyperbilirubinaemia	
Physiological	Mononucleosis
Breast milk	Crigler–Najjar syndrome
Haemolytic (ABO incompatibility)	Reye syndrome, Metabolic
Drug-induced jaundice	Wilson disease
Gilbert's syndrome	Polycythaemia
Direct hyperbilirubinaemia	Malaria
Infectious Hepatitis	Cystic fibrosis
Autoimmune hepatitis	Leptospirosis
Biliary atresia	Alagille syndrome
Drug-induced hepatitis	Hypothyroidism
Metabolic hepatitis	Alpha-1 antitrypsin deficiency
	Q fever
	Niemann-Pick disease

Misdiagnosis is due:

1st mistake: failing to establish conditions mimicking jaundice (pseudo-jaundice).

2nd mistake: failing to establish diagnostic criteria of physiological jaundice.

3rd mistake: failing to set up diagnostic criteria of pathological jaundice during neonatal period.

4th mistake: failing to differentiate the main causes of childhood jaundice.

5th mistake: forgetting about Gilbert's syndrome in the differential diagnosis of hyperbilirubinaemia.

6th mistake: ignoring autoimmune hepatitis and other forms of hepatitis.

1. Conditions that Mimic Jaundice:

   - Jaundice should be differentiated from xanthochromia (carotenaemia), which is due to carotene deposits in the skin and increased beta-carotene level in the blood.
   - Carotenaemia is characterised by yellow pigmentation of the skin caused by prolonged and excessive consumption of carotene-rich diet such as carrots and sweet potatoes.
   - It is a harmless condition but it can lead to a mistaken diagnosis of jaundice. Normal white sclerae is an important diagnostic clue against the presence of jaundice. Normal serum bilirubin confirms the diagnosis.

2. Physiological Jaundice

   - Physiologic jaundice occurs in most neonates during the first week of life, peaking at 6–8 mg/dl by 3 days of life. Premature infants have a higher level of hyperbilirubinaemia peaking on the fifth day of life.
   - It is not a disease, it is not present in the first 24 h and it is always an indirect hyperbilirubinaemia.
   - Breast milk jaundice is nothing else than physiologic jaundice, which peaks by 5–15 days of life, and usually disappears by the third week of life. It occurs in about 10% of breast-fed babies. Mothers should be encouraged to continue breast feeding.
   - Diagnosis of physiological and breast milk jaundice is by eliminating other causes of jaundice, the infant is in good health, feeding well and gaining weight adequately.

3. Criteria for Non-Physiological Jaundice

   - Clinical jaundice prior to 24 h of age.
   - Total serum bilirubin level >15 mg/dl in a formula-fed and >17 mg/dl in breast-fed term infant.

- Total serum bilirubin levels increasing by >5 mg/dl per day.
- A direct bilirubin more than 25 μmol/L (or 15% of the total bilirubin).
- Clinical jaundice persisting after 8 days in a term infant or after 14 days in a premature infant.
- Associated with unwell-appearing, lethargy, poor feeding.

4. Main Causes of Pathological Jaundice
   Haemolytic Anaemia

- Haemolytic anaemia includes ABO and Rh-incompatibility, glucose-6-phosphate dehydrogenase (G-6PD) deficiency and hereditary spherocytosis.
- Clinical jaundice usually appears in the first 24 h after the birth.
- Diagnostic confirmation is by the findings of blood group, Rh types, packed cell volume (PCV), Hb, with reticulocytosis and positive Coombs test.

   Hepatocellular Diseases

- Direct-reacting bilirubin is water-soluble, and therefore it does not damage the brain tissue to cause kernicterus. It is however associated with serious diseases, such as congenital hepatitis and biliary atresia.
- A direct bilirubin more than 25 μmol/L (or 15% of the total bilirubin) indicates serious disease and is never physiologic. Causes include neonatal hepatitis secondary to congenital infection (rubella, CMV, toxoplasmosis) or biliary atresia.
- In hepatocellular disease, there is a disproportional increase of alanine aminotransferase (ALT) and aspartate aminotransferase (AST) compared to alkaline phosphatase increase; whereas in cholestatic diseases it is the opposite. ALT is present in the liver, hence more specific than AST which is present in other organs.

Biliary Atresia

- Children with biliary atresia are usually healthy looking and indistinguishable from those with physiological jaundice during the first two weeks.
- When jaundice lasts more than 2 weeks, direct bilirubin should always be measured. The presence of pale chalky or acholic stools (stool colour cards) and/or dark urine that stains the nappy are suggestive of biliary atresia.
- It is urgent to refer an infant with direct hyperbilirubinaemia before irreversible damage to the liver is done. The Kasai operation (portoenterostomy) is successful (>90%) if performed before 8 weeks of life. Without Kasai operation (to drain bile from the liver into the intestines) or liver transplantation, liver failure ensues within a year and death within 2 years.

5. Diagnostic Criteria of Gilbert's Syndrome (Table 6.4)

6. Differential Diagnosis of Hepatitis
   After the neonatal period, infection remains the most common cause of jaundice worldwide. The incidence of hepatitis A (HA) has declined significantly in developed countries. Table 6.5 facilitates the differential diagnosis of jaundice caused by hepatitis.

TABLE 6.4 Diagnostic criteria of Gilbert's syndrome

- Gilbert's syndrome is a common (affecting 8–9% of the population) recessive inherited condition caused by mutations to the UGT1A1 gene. Uridine-diphosphoglucuronate glucuronosyl-transferase levels are reduced
- The syndrome is characterised by a mild rise of indirect hyperbilirubinaemia (not exceeding 102 micromol/L = <6 mg/dL) in the absence of hepatocellular injury or haemolysis
- It is a benign condition and patients are usually asymptomatic but may present with an episode of abdominal pain. Jaundice becomes apparent during fasting, sleep deprivation or stress

TABLE 6.5 Differential diagnosis of the most common causes of hepatitis in older children

Condition	Presentation	Diagnostic features
Autoimmune hepatitis	Acute, acute fulminant hepatitis, or asymptomatic. Symptoms of acute hepatitis as with viral hepatitis (see below)	• Auto-antibodies (ANA, SMA) • Presence of high serum AST and ALT • Hypergammaglobulinaemia • Negative IgM anti-HAV, HBsAg, HBV DNA, HCV RNA • Histological confirmation of hepatitis • Other diagnoses (e.g. viral hepatitis) are excluded
Viral Hepatitis (A, B, C, D, E)	80% of cases: asymptomatic. Presentation includes fever, malaise, nausea, anorexia, abdominal pain, dark urine & acholic stools. Signs include hepatosplenomegaly, hepatic tenderness.	• Jaundice occurs in 1:10 children with hepatitis A, 1 in 4 with hepatitis B, and 1 in 3 in hepatitis C • Abnormal LFT, with direct (conjugated) hyperbilirubinaemia, high AST, ALT, GGT, IgM anti-HA for each virus

(continued)

TABLE 6.5 (continued)

Condition	Presentation	Diagnostic features
Drug-induced hepatitis (Antibiotics, NSAIDs, some herbal medicine)	As a hepatitis with jaundice (see viral hepatitis)	• Diagnosis of exclusion • Abnormal LFT, negative IgM for viruses • Autoantibodies • History of drug intake
Mononucleosis	Fever, Pharyngitis, lymphadenopathy, hepato-splenomegaly	• Abnormal LFT(e.g. AST & ALT, prothrombin) • Atypical lymphocytes • Positive EBV-IgM & Monospot
Metabolic liver diseases, e.g. Glycogen storage, haemochromatosis, porphyria, Wilson disease	Failure to thrive, lethargy, pruritis. Signs include hepatomegaly	• Abnormal LFTs with elevated direct hyperbilirubiaemia, hypoalbuminaemia • High coper in urine, low ceruloplasmin (for Wilson disease)

LFT liver function tests, *AST* aspartate transaminase, *ALT* alanine transaminase, *HAV* hepatitis A virus, *HBsAg* hepatitis B surface antigen, *GGT* gamma-glutamyl transpeptide, *NSAIDs* Non-steroidal anti-inflammatory drugs

Further Reading

Hijaz NM, Friesen CA. Managing acute abdominal pain in pediatric patients: current perspectives. Pediatr Health Med Ther. 2017;8:83–91.

Yang WC, Chen CY, Wu HP. Etiology of non-traumatic acute abdomen in pediatric emergency departments. World J Clin Cases. 2013;1(9):276–84.

Horst S, Shelby G, Anderson J, et al. Predicting persistence of functional abdominal pain from childhood into young adulthood. Clin Gastroenterol Hepatol. 2014;12(12):2026–32.

Korterink JJ, Diederson K, Benninga MA, et al. Epidemiology of pediatric functional abdominal pain disorders: a meta-analysis. PLoS One. 2015;10(5):e0126982.

Brusafero A, Farinelli E, Zenzeri L, et al. The management of paediatric functional abdominal pain disorders: latest evidence. Paediatr Drugs. 2018;20(3):235–47.

da Jesus LE, Cestari AB, da Silva OC, et al. Pathologic aerophagia: a rare case of chronic abdominal distension. Rev Paul Pediatr. 2015;33(3):371–5.

Mukhopadhyay B, Mukhopadhyay M, Mondal KC, et al. Hirschsprung's disease in neonates with special reference to Calretinin immunohistochemistry. J Clin Diagn Res. 2015;9(7):EC06–9.

Greggoria GV, Gonzales MM, Dans LF, et al. Polymer-based oral rehydration solution for treating acute watery diarrhoea. Cochrane Database Syst Rev. 2016;12:CD006519.

Carter E, Bryce J, Perin J, et al. Harmful practices in the management of childhood diarrhoea in low- and middle income countries: a systematic review. BMC Public Health. 2015;15:788.

Romano C, Oliva S, Martellosi S, et al. Pediatric gastrointestinal bleeding: perspective from the Italian Society of Pediatric Gastroenterology. World J Gastroenterol. 2017;23(8):1328–37.

Wang KS. Newborn screening for biliary atresia. Pediatrics. 2015;136(6):e1663–9.

Chen H, Wu S, Hsu S, et al. Jaundice revisited: recent advances in the diagnosis and treatment of inherited cholestatic liver diseases. J Biomed Sci. 2018;25:75.

Chapter 7
Neurology

7.1 Neonatal Seizures

Introduction/Core Messages

- Neonatal seizure is a paroxysmal alteration in neurological function, i.e. behavioural, motor and/or autonomic function. An EEG definition involves a clear ictal event of suddenly repetitive, evolving stereotyped waveforms lasting minimum ictal duration of 10 sec in infants younger than 28 days.
- Seizures are common in paediatric population occurring in 5–7% of children older than neonates. Neonates have the highest incidence of seizures: in pre-terms it is 4–9% and in term infants it is 0.1–0.4%.
- Neonates have the highest risk of seizures compared to older children because of the immaturity of inhibitory neuro-transmission and increased susceptibility to large cerebral and systemic insults.
- The usual well-known tonic-clonic seizures seen in older children are not seen in neonates: Their seizures are mainly oral, e.g. chewing, lip smacking, eye jerks or apnoea.

© Springer Nature Switzerland AG 2021   137
A. S. El-Radhi, *Avoiding Misdiagnosis in Pediatric Practice*,
In Clinical Practice, https://doi.org/10.1007/978-3-030-41750-5_7

- The recognition of neonatal seizures is often difficult and therefore both over- and under-diagnosis may occur. Neonates frequently exhibit abnormal non-epileptic involuntary movements that may be mistaken for seizures. Even normal movements may also be considered as seizures. For these cases, continuous video-EEG monitoring is the gold standard for diagnosing epileptic seizures.
- As neonatal seizures differ in aetiologies and presentation from those in older children, the two are separately presented.

Differential Diagnosis

Common	Rare
Hypoxic-ischaemic encephalopathy (HIE)	Mitochondrial disease
Cerebral haemorrhage	Fifth-day seizure
Metabolic (e.g. hypoglycaemia, hypocalcaemia)	Inborn errors of metabolism
Infection (e.g. meningitis)	Pyridoxine-dependency
Developmental/malformation	
Neonatal withdrawal syndrome	

Misdiagnosis is due to:

1st mistake: failing to recognise neonatal seizures.

2nd mistake: not considering conditions mimicking seizures.

3rd mistake: failing to determine the underlying causes of neonatal seizures.

1. Recognising Neonatal Seizures
   - Recognition of seizures depends on a detailed history, excluding conditions mimicking seizures, and investigation to confirm the clinical findings.
   - Seizures are recognised by the following features:
     - Description of the event by a witness. Smartphone video helps diagnosing epilepsy.

- A search in the history for risk factors including maternal drug history, inherited diseases, history of asphyxia and Apgar score.
- Physical examination should focus on the general appearance, level of consciousness, i.e. any degree of drowsiness or alternatively irritability, noticing any irregular respiration pattern or fluctuating body temperature.

- Patterns of seizures include:
  - Subtle seizures, e.g. repetitive blinking, fluttering, fixation or deviation upwards or downwards of the eyes. Tonic posturing of a limb, rowing or pedalling. Episodic apnoea, tonic (generalized or focal).
  - Focal or multifocal clonic jerks that are not associated with loss of consciousness.
  - Myoclonia (focal or multi -focal), single or multiple slow jerks of the limbs that are usually associated with diffuse CNS abnormalities; prognosis is poor.

2. Conditions that Mimic Seizures
  - Jitteriness: occurring frequently in babies aged few hours to few weeks, and is characterised by:

    - Fast rhythmic movements of the limbs that are abnormal in appearance but are non-epileptic and often mistaken for seizures leading to inappropriate investigation and treatment.
    - Absence of gaze or eye movements, cyanosis, bradycardia, tachycardia, decreased oxygen saturation or increased blood pressure.
    - Stretching the joint can provoke jitteriness in contrast to the spontaneous occurrence of seizures.
    - Cessation of jitteriness with gentle restraint or passive flexion of a limb.
    - Video EEG shows normal record.

  - Infants of diabetic mothers are frequently jittery even with normal blood sugar and calcium levels.
  - Benign neonatal sleep myoclonus: Face is never involved, facial colour normal. Cessation usually aged 3–6 m. EEG is normal.

- Myoclonus jerks consist of sudden brief bursts of myoclonia occurring mainly while the child is awake. Development and EEG are normal.

Investigations for Neonatal Seizures

- Blood for blood glucose, calcium, magnesium, urea and electrolytes, bicarbonate, blood culture, CRP. Serum amino acids, ammonia, lactate, pyruvate, organic acids, pH, ketones, liver function tests, fatty acids are usually performed when clinically indicated.
- CSF for analysis and culture.
- Cranial ultrasonography, possibly CT scan or MRI.
- EEG recording: Ictal and inter-ictal EEG abnormalities are non-specific showing sharp, and rarely, spike forms, focal or multi-focal. Gross abnormalities such as burst-suppression pattern carry a very bad prognosis.

3. The Main Causes of Neonatal Seizures
   Hypoxic-Ischaemic Encephalopathy (HIE)

- HIE is the most important consequence of perinatal asphyxia, a frequent cause of seizure (within 12–24 h of birth) and a common cause of later epilepsy.
- Seizures, including subclinical seizures, due to HIE are very common (about 25–50%). There is evidence that seizures exacerbate ischaemic brain injury. Therapeutical hypothermia has been used to reduce this injury and neurological morbidities.
- Diagnostic criteria include abnormal foetal heart rate pattern, low Apgar scores at birth, jitteriness, lethargy, poor feeding and seizures (tonic and multifocal seizures).
- Continuous video-EEG monitoring is recommended for at least 24 hours.

Ischaemic Stroke

- This is the second most common cause of neonatal seizures after HIE. Seizures typically occur in older age than they do with HIE (24–48 hours).

- Typical presentation is focal seizure often associated with intracranial haemorrhage.

Intracranial Haemorrhage (ICH)

- ICH occurs in 20% to more than 40% in infants with birthweights of <1.5 kg.
- Isolated intraventricular haemorrhage (IVH) is rarely associated with neonatal seizures unless the IVH is large or there is in addition parenchymal haemorrhage.

CNS Infections

- Although CNS infections during the first few days of life represent only 5% of cases of neonatal seizures, prompt treatment is essential to minimise the damage effects on the CNS.
- Seizures due to CNS infections usually persist longer than with HIE or intracranial haemorrhage due to persistent inflammation.
- Symptoms and signs of CNS infections are shown in (Table 7.1).

TABLE 7.1 Symptoms and signs of a child with serious bacterial infection including meningitis

General	Reduced activity, weak cry, poor eye contact
Body temperature	Instability, fever, hypothermia
Signs of shock	Clammy, mottled skin, prolonged CRT >2–3 s
Respiratory	Apnoea, tachypnoea, shallow respiration, grunting
Gastrointestinal	Poor feeding, vomiting, abdominal distension, diarrhoea
CNS	Drowsiness, sometimes alternating with irritability, bulging fontanelle, neck stiffness is usually absent

CRT Capillary refill time

Metabolic Causes

- Hypoglycaemia: premature, small for date babies, babies with sepsis or asphyxia are at risk of hypoglycaemia and seizures.
- Hypocalcaemia is the second most common cause of neonatal seizures caused by prematurity, sepsis, infants of mothers with diabetes. Seizure types include clonus and jitteriness. Seizures occurring after the first week are usually focal with an EEG showing focal abnormalities.
- Other metabolic problems include hyponatraemia, pyridoxine deficiency and amino acid metabolism disorders.

7.2   Seizures in Older Children (Epilepsy)

Introduction/Core Messages
- Febrile seizures (FS) are the most common cause of seizures occurring in 3–4%, followed by epileptic seizure occurring in 1%.
- Although the diagnosis of seizures depends almost entirely on the history of eyewitnesses (parents, observer), but they are often incapable of recognising subtle events.
- A diagnosis of epilepsy should carefully be considered as 20–40% of patients diagnosed as having epilepsy do not actually have epilepsy. A wrongly made diagnosis of epilepsy may restrict the child's activities including leisure activity, education and employment. In addition to the use of anti-epileptic drugs (AEDs), which can cause adverse features.
- On the other hand, if the diagnosis of epilepsy is not made (e.g. epilepsy wrongly diagnosed as cardiac syncope), the patient is denied the necessary treatment for an epileptic patient, and possibly receiving harmful treatment as a patient with syncope.
- Epileptic seizures have to be differentiated from non-epileptic seizures (e.g. pseudo-seizure, breath

holding attacks) defined as motor activity or behaviour that resemble epileptic seizures but without abnormal/ excessive discharges of neurons.

- Misdiagnosis of epilepsy is common and due to:

  - Not obtaining a proper history as the diagnosis is mainly based on the history.
  - Atypical presentations of epilepsy if they manifest as psychiatric symptoms.
  - Many clinicians do not have sufficient knowledge of the clinical features of epilepsy and non-epileptic seizure.
  - A large list of differential diagnosis which mimic epileptic seizures.
  - EEG may lead to a misdiagnosis.

Common	Rare
Febrile seizure	Cerebral tumours
Epilepsy (generalised and partial)	Cerebral haemorrhage
Metabolic (e.g. Hypoglycaemia)	Drug-induced
Infection (e.g. meningitis)	
Psychogenic non-epileptic seizures	
Intra-cranial tumour	

Misdiagnosis of epilepsy is common due to:

1st mistake: failing to establish the diagnosis of epilepsy.

2nd mistake: failing to differentiate syncope from epilepsy.

3rd mistake: failing to differentiate pseudo-seizure (Psychogenic) from true epilepsy.

4th mistake: failing to distinguish febrile seizures from epileptic seizures.

5th mistake: failing to differentiate other less common conditions mimicking seizures.

6th mistake: misleading EEG diagnosis.

1. Diagnosing Epilepsy

As many as 20–40% of patients diagnosed as having epilepsy do not have actually epilepsy. The diagnosis of epilepsy is based on certain clinical criteria, excluding events mimicking seizures and by the use of an EEG.

- Epilepsy is defined in the year 2014 by ILAE (International League Against Epilepsy) as one of the following: 1) at least two unprovoked or reflex seizures occurring > 24hours apart; 2) one unprovoked or reflex seizure and a probability of further seizures occurring over the next 10 years; 3) a diagnosis of an epileptic syndrome. There are currently around 30 epileptic syndromes.
- The recognition of epileptic seizures is almost always dependent on obtaining a detailed history so that the diagnosis is rapidly established. Diagnostic delays (an interval of > 1 month from the seizure onset) are associated with detrimental impact on the child's cognitive development.
- Epilepsy is recently classified as generalised, implying a bilateral cerebral hemispheric involvement, with 6 subtypes (including tonic-clonic, absence and myoclonia seizures), and focal, implying one hemispheric involvement with 3 subtypes.
- The diagnosis of epileptic seizures should only be made by experienced professionals such as paediatricians with special interest in epilepsy or paediatric neurologists. If the diagnosis remains uncertain from the history, it is appropriate to await further episodes.

2. Differentiating Syncope from Epilepsy
- Syncope is a very common condition affecting about 40% of the population. It is the most frequent cause of misdiagnosis in epilepsy as both conditions are associated with transient loss of consciousness/awareness and abnormal movements. Syncope and epilepsy may coexist in about 20% of cases.

- Syncope is defined as a transient (lasting no longer than 20 s), self-limited loss of consciousness with an inability to maintain postural tone that is followed by spontaneous recovery. The recovery is rapid with immediate restoration of appropriate behaviour and orientation. There may be a prodromal sensation of warmth, light-headedness, sweating and facial pallor. Other possible features include tonic-clonic or myoclonic jerking, oral automatism but urine incontinence or tongue biting is unusual. If tongue biting occurs it is usually on the tip of the tongue only.
- The diagnosis of syncope is supported by Tilt-Table Testing (the standard diagnostic testing) and typical decrease in systolic BP of >20 mm Hg and/or a decrease in diastolic of >10 mm Hg within 3 minutes of standing.
- Cardiac causes of syncope should always be considered, particularly if the syncope occurs during exertion, when supine or in association with palpitation, chest discomfort, breathlessness, or known to have ECG abnormalities such as QTc interval > 460 ms or prolonged PR interval.
- One specific type of syncope is POTS (Postural Tachycardia Syndrome) that has recently been increasingly recognised. POTS is a form of orthostatic intolerance. Diagnostic criteria are:

    - Increase HR > 40 bpm within a min of standing from a supine position
    - Associated symptoms (palpitation, light-headedness, chest discomfort, dyspnoea, nausea, general weakness) that appear in upright position and that improve with recumbence
    - The tachycardia is not associated with orthostatic hypotension
    - Chronicity of the symptoms > 6 months

3. Psychogenic Non-Epileptic Seizures (Pseudo-seizures)
    Diagnosis is characterised by:

- Seizure occurs typically at 10–18 years of age, more in females, and often in the presence of an audience.
- Seizures are bizarre, unusual muscle contracture, with pelvic thrusting and rolling movements.
- Absence of cyanosis, tongue biting, urinary incontinence or injury.
- Gradual onset and waxing and waning during the episode, with rapid recovery.
- Less stereotyped and of briefer duration compared with epileptic seizures.
- No genuine loss of consciousness or post-ictal drowsiness.
- Normal serum prolactin (raised in true epilepsy).
- Normal EEG.

4. Febrile Seizure (FS):

- This is the most common cause of seizures occurring between 6 months to 5 years in a neurologically normal child. Family history of FS is common.
- Fever is always present at onset; i.e. absence of fever excludes FS.
- Usually the child is well prior to onset.
- Duration of seizure and unconsciousness is usually brief, and recovery is rapid.
- The child is well after the seizure, without signs of meningitis such as neck stiffness or bulging fontanelle.

5. Conditions Mimicking Epileptic Seizures

Breath holding	• See Table 7.2 to differentiate breath holding from epilepsy
Narcolepsy	• Narcolepsy is characterised by recurring daytime sleepiness, often associated with disrupted sleep at night, cataplexy (loss of muscle control when, for example, laughing), sleep paralysis and hypnagogic phenomenon (auditory or visual illusion or hallucination when falling asleep)
Benign paroxysmal vertigo	• Attacks occur without warning and resolve spontaneously • Attacks occur mainly in toddlers • After a few seconds there is a sudden onset of pallor, unsteadiness, crying for help, clinging to his mother or refusing to walk, often with vomiting and horizontal nystagmus • Episodes may last up to 30 sec and recur in days or weeks
The long QT-syndrome	• Is either autosomal dominant inherited (Romano–Ward syndrome), autosomal recessive (Jervell–Lange-Nelson syndrome) or acquired (myocarditis or electrolyte disturbance). It is an important cause of loss of consciousness and may mimic epilepsy. Child may recover immediately after the episode or die during the event. A heart rate-corrected QT-interval > 470 milliseconds supports the diagnosis, whereas a QT-interval > 440 milliseconds is suspicious
Night terror	• Parents of children with night terrors are often woken by piercing scream, child looks flushed, frightened and agitated, and is not easily aroused • The child cannot recall the event next morning

TABLE 7.2 Differential diagnosis between breath holding and epileptic seizure

---

- Excluding febrile seizures, epileptic seizures are uncommon and 10 times less common (0.5%) than breath holding (5%)

- Epilepsy occurs at any age; the age of children with breath holding is usually 1–3 years

- Cyanosis in breath holding occurs first before the onset of subsequent seizure while cyanosis occurs after the onset of epileptic seizure

- Breath holding spells are nearly always stereotyped (as above), epileptic seizures are unpredictable in the way they occur

- Recovery is fast in breath holding (1–2 min) while the recovery in seizure takes longer duration

- There is no post-ictal phase in breath holding in contrast to seizures

- The EEG is normal in breath holding, and likely abnormal in epilepsy

---

6. Misleading EEG Diagnosis

- EEG is a useful investigation in seizure disorders including diagnosing absence seizure (spike-wave), non-convulsive status epilepticus, classifying the specific epilepsy syndrome and differentiating between primary and secondarily generalised seizures.

- However, EEG diagnosis may be misleading as it lacks both sensitivity and specificity. Many children with epilepsy will have a normal EEG obtained from a single inter-ictal EEG, and 5% of healthy children without epilepsy have epileptiform EEG discharges. Over-interpretation of the EEG is an important cause of misdiagnosis as a number of benign variant patterns not related to epilepsy are often considered epileptiform.

- The yield of inter-ictal epileptiform discharges in the routine outpatient EEG is low, around 28% only.

- EEG has limited diagnostic value in identifying certain types of epilepsy such as occipital lobe epilepsy.

- Although a prolonged (hours and days) EEG monitoring or video-EEG recoding to obtain an ictal event is very helpful diagnostically, the technique is available only in specialised centres.
- Although sleep EEG is a very effective diagnostic tool as 67% of generalised epileptiform discharges occur in NREM sleep phase, this is an expensive test and may require putting the child to sleep.

7.3   Headache

Introduction/Core Messages
- This is a very common problem, occurring in about 50% of children aged 7 years and 80% of children aged 15 years. Although most causes of headaches in children are benign, it is essential to consider an underlying systemic disease.
- Infants or toddlers with headache may present with irritability, unwillingness to play, crying while holding the head or vomiting.
- Alternating hemiplegia may be the first sign of later migraine. Frequent vasoconstriction causing hemiplegia causes ischaemia which may lead to cerebral injury and developmental delay later on.
- Cluster headache is rare in children and is characterised by severe, unilateral pain affecting the orbital and supra-orbital pain. Associated features include conjunctival injection, lacrimal and nasal congestion and facial sweating. The pain lasts 15–180 min and occurs several times daily in series over weeks or months separated by remission of months or years.
- A headache worse in the morning, which increases with stooping or straining suggests raised intracranial pressure.

- Benign ICP is characterised by symptoms of raised ICP (e.g. headaches, vomiting and papilloedema) with normal level of consciousness, CSF and ventricular size (as evident by CT scan or MRI). Focal neurological signs are absent. An urgent same-day referral to hospital is required to exclude brain tumour.
- Neuro-imaging is not indicated on a routine basis in children with recurrent headaches and normal physical examination. It is indicated with abnormal neurological examination, progressive headaches or co-existing seizure. Common and rare causes of headache are listed below.

Differential Diagnosis

Common	Rare
Common viral infections	Eye strain
Migraine	Cluster headaches
Tension headaches	Head injury
Increased ICP due to tumour	Hypertension
	Sinusitis

Misdiagnosis is due to:

1st Mistake: Failing to establish the diagnosis of migraine.

2nd Mistake: Failing to consider migraine variants.

3rd Mistake: Failing to differentiate migraine from tension headaches.

4th Mistake: Failing to differentiating functional from structural-related headaches.

1. Diagnosis of Migraine

Migraine without aura (common migraine), the most common type of migraine, is defined in Table 7.3. Criteria for diagnosing migraine with aura (classical migraine) are defined in Table 7.4. Aura occurs in about 20% of cases before the onset of migraine and lasts 20–60 min. It manifests as a sensory sensation that includes flashes of light, blurry vision and tingling in the hand or face.

TABLE 7.3 Criteria for diagnosing migraine without aura

- >5 attacks fulfilling the following criteria:

- Headache lasting 1–72 h

- Headache has at least 2 of the following 4 criteria:

  - Bilateral or unilateral location

  - Pulsating quality

  - Moderate to severe pain intensity

  - Aggravated by physical activities e.g. climbing stairs

- At least 1 of the following accompanies headache:

  - Nausea and/or vomiting

  - Photophobia and phonophobia

TABLE 7.4 Criteria for diagnosing migraine with aura

At least 2 attacks showing at least 3 of the 4 following criteria:

- One or more reversible aura symptoms

- At least 1 aura develops gradually > 4 min

- No aura symptoms lasting > 1 h

- Headache follows aura with a free interval of <1 h but may begin before or may simultaneously with aura

2. Diagnosis of Migraine Variants

   Migraine variants are common and should be differentiated from migraine (Table 7.5).

3. To Differentiate Tension Headache from Migraine

   - Distinguishing migraine from tension-type headache is essential because the aetiology and management are different (Table 7.6).
   - It is simple to differentiate the two most common causes of headaches. Migraine disrupts the child's activity, whereas tension headache does not.

TABLE 7.5 Clinical features of migraine variants

Abdominal migraine	• Episodic abdominal pain, moderate to severe, typically peri-umbilical, often associated headache • Accompanied nausea with or without vomiting, pallor • Usually lasts few hours, range 1–72 h, is terminated by sleep • Typical age 4–8 years, very rarely before 2 years • Strong family history of migraine
Cyclic vomiting	• Bouts of vomiting that may last hours or days, often associated with headache • Two previous episodes in the past 6 months are needed to make the diagnosis • Triggers include infections, stress or the use of cannabinoid
Ophthalmic migraine	• Unilateral eye pain and 3rd nerve palsy with ptosis, papillary dilatation and external eye deviation
Basilar artery migraine	• Ataxia, vertigo, diplopia, vomiting, dysarthria, weakness, syncope, scotoma or transient blindness • With these symptoms, posterior fossa lesions (e.g. tumour) needs to be excluded
Acute confusional state	• Change in orientation, personality or behaviour (restless, hyperactive) • Confusion may last minutes to hours • It may occur after minor head trauma
Benign paroxysmal Vertigo of childhood	• Sudden unsteadiness with nystagmus and vomiting occurring typically in toddlers (median age 18 months). Child appears frightened and pale • The spell lasts minutes and often occurs in clusters over several days, then subsiding for weeks or months • Normal neurological examination and vestibular function • Typically there is a family history of migraine and the children will develop typical migraine in the future

(continued)

Table 7.5 (continued)

Paroxysmal torticollis of infancy	• These benign and recurrent episodes of head tilt associated with pallor, agitation, vomiting and ataxia. The tilt may alternate from side to side • The initial paroxysms typically affect infancy; spontaneous remission occurs aged 2–3 years. Episode may last minutes to days • Cerebellum or vestibulo-cerebellar pathways are probably involved. Abnormalities of the cervical vertebrae (e.g. dislocation) or posterior fossa tumour should be considered, particularly if the episodes are prolonged

Table 7.6 Diagnostic criteria of tension-type of headaches

• Headache lasting 30 min to 7 days

• At least 2 of the following pain characteristics

– Pressing or tightening (not pulsating)

– Mild or moderate intensity

– Bilateral location

– No aggravation by physical activities

• In addition

– No nausea or vomiting

– No photophobia or phonophobia

– No evidence of structural or metabolic disease

4. Headaches Caused by Increased ICP

• Headaches are common in children with intracranial tumours, occurring in over 50%. They are usually associated with other symptoms and signs of increased intracranial pressure (ICP) but can be the only symptom.

• Headaches caused by ICP may resemble migraine or tension-type headaches, particularly at the onset of symptoms.

• Symptoms that require urgent attention and the differential diagnosis of these symptoms are shown in Table 7.7.

TABLE 7.7 Differential diagnosis of conditions that suggest an increased ICP

Condition	Characteristic features
• Brain neoplasm	Early morning headache with or without vomiting, without nausea, worsening or occipital headache, seizures, and/or personality changes
• Basilar migraine	Presenting with vertigo, diplopia, blurred vision and ataxia. (It should be differentiated from posterior fossa tumour)
• Benign ICP	Is characterised by increased ICP (e.g. headaches, vomiting and papilloedema) with normal CSF and ventricular size. Focal neurological signs are absent

7.4   Coma

Introduction/Core Messages
- Impaired levels of consciousness are associated with significant mortality. Clinicians rely on scores such as Glasgow Coma Scale (GCS) to evaluate levels of consciousness and to identify children who need further intervention.
- Children have a reduced levels of consciousness (coma) with GCS score <15 (infancy) or <14 (older children). A CT scan is usually required with these scores.
- AVPU (A=Alert, V=respond to Voice, P=to Pain or U=unresponsive) is a simple scale that may be used easily at the site of injury. A child who do well on AVPU have an equivalent score >14–15 on GCS.

Differential Diagnosis

Common	Rare
Seizures	
Head injury	Cerebral malaria
Toxins/poisoning/medication	Infection (meningitis)

Common	Rare
Intracranial infection	Urea cycle disorder
	Diabetic ketoacidosis (DKA)/ hypoglycaemia
	Hysteria
	Reye syndrome
	Intracranial haemorrhage (e.g. stroke)

Misdiagnosis is due:

1. Mistake: Failing to define the most common causes of central nervous system (CNS) infections.
2. Mistake: Failing to differentiate cranial causes of CNS infections that may lead to coma.
3. Mistake: Failing to recognise common non-cranial causes that may lead to coma.

1. Definitions of CNS Infections (Table 7.8)

   - The CNS is defined by the brain (cerebrum and cerebellum), spine, optic nerves and their covering membranes.
   - Infections of the CSF are medical emergencies requiring urgent action.
   - The infection compromises 3 main categories: meningitis, encephalitis and abscess, which are generally result from blood-borne spread microorganisms: S pneumoniae, N meningitides, and H influenzae.
   - Normal CSF in neonates may contain up to 25–30 white cells, with up to 60% neutrophils. Few days later, the number of white cells in the CSF decreased to 8–9. In older children, the CSF contains less than 4–5 white cells/mm^3, usually lymphocytes.

2. CNS Infections that may Lead to Coma
   - Neonatal meningitis (see also section Seizures above) manifests as lethargy, irritability, poor feeding, thermal instability, respiratory distress apnoea, seizures.
   - Older children present with:

TABLE 7.8 Definitions of meningitis, meningococcal disease and encephalitis

- Confirmed meningitis: isolation of bacteria from CSF, blood or DNA detection through PCR from a patient with a CSF pleocytosis of white cells >10 cells/mm3. In neonates a pleocytosis of ≥ 20 white cells is accepted. Diagnosis is also accepted in case of postmortem diagnosis

- Probable meningitis: the presence of clinical symptoms and signs of bacterial meningitis in the absence of laboratory confirmation

- Meningococcal disease: a clinical condition caused by Neisseria meningitidis with purulent conjunctivitis, septic arthritis, and septicaemia with or without meningitis

- Aseptic meningitis: the presence of CSF white cell count >10 cells/mm³; CSF is negative for bacterial culture, occurring usually in summer months. Viruses are most common causes

- Encephalitis: an inflammation of the parenchymal tissue of the brain caused by an infection producing varying degrees of impaired consciousness

---

- – Non-specific early symptoms (in the first 4–6 h) are fever, irritability and decreased appetite. This is followed (at a median time of 8h) by early symptoms of sepsis: leg pain, abnormal skin colour, and cold hands and feet. Classic meningitis symptoms appear later (13–22 h): purpuric rash, impaired consciousness and meningism.
  – Fever, vomiting headache.
  – Meningococcal septicaemia.
  – Febrile convulsive status epilepticus.

- TB meningitis often occurs within 6 months of the initial TB infection following haematogenous dissemination or a rupture of a subependymal focus into subarachnoid space. Fever is the most common presenting symptom, and meningism (e.g. neck stiffness) is the most common finding at presentation. The incidence is highest in children aged 1–5 years. The three recognized stages are:

- Conscious with non-specific symptoms (fever, night sweats, anorexia, weight loss, fatigue) and no neurological signs.
- Onset of neurological signs: headache, confusion, drowsiness, neck stiffness.
- Stupor, deepening coma, focal neurological signs.

• Herpes simplex infection (HSI) should be suspected clinically in a child with reduced conscious level if one or more of the following 4 are present:

- Focal neurological signs.
- Fluctuating conscious level for 6 hours or more.
- Contact with herpetic lesions.
- No obvious clinical signs pointing towards the cause.

• Intracranial Abscess should be suspected in a child with a reduced conscious level with:

- Focal neurological signs +/- clinical signs of sepsis.
- Signs of increased ICP.
- Diagnosis is confirmed by imaging.

3. Non-Intracranial Causes of Coma.

• Sepsis/septic shock. Sepsis is defined as the systemic response to an infection, and is characterised by:

- A body temperature of >38.0°C or <35.5°C.
- Tachycardia and tachypnoea.
- A rise in WBC of >15.000 or a fall of WBC <5.000, or if there is non-blanching petechial or purpuric skin rash.

• Circulatory shock is diagnosed if one or more of the following signs are present:

- Mottled/cool extremities.
- Diminished peripheral pulse.
- Systolic blood pressure <5th % for age.
- Capillary refill time >2 sec.
- Urine output < 1ml/kg/h.

• Other conditions that may cause coma include trauma, metabolic disorders (e.g. hypoglycaemia, hypocalcaemia, hyperammonaemia), and poisoning.

7.5   Tremor

Introduction/Core Messages

- Tremor is an involuntary, rhythmic oscillatory movement that can be physiological and pathological. Tremor is the most common movement disorder in clinical practice. Cerebello-thalamo-cortical pathway is involved in almost all pathological tremor.
- Tremor may occur at rest or in action. Resting tremor is present when the child sits with his/her arms resting without voluntary movement. Action tremor is subdivided into postural (an arm maintaining a position against gravity) and kinetic which is associated with voluntary movement. Intentional tremor is characterised by an increase of tremor amplitude as the target is approached. This can be demonstrated by finger-nose-finger test.
- Jitteriness, a rhythmic tremor of equal amplitude, is very common in healthy neonates, particularly premature infants and when babies are crying.
- Misdiagnosis of tremor is common because clinicians frequently overlook diagnostic features of each type of tremor as well as overlook additional neurological signs that are associated with this symptom.

Differential Diagnosis

Common	Rare
Physiological tremor	Cerebral palsy
Essential tremor (autosomal dominant)	Acute confusional state
Anxiety	Hyperthyroidism
Medications (e.g. β-2 agonists for asthma)	Wilson's disease

Common	Rare
	Juvenile Parkinson's disease
	Spinocerebellar ataxia
	Acute intermittent porphyria

Misdiagnosis is due to:

1st Mistake: Failing to recognise physiological tremor.

2nd Mistake: Failing to differentiate tremor from other movement disorders (e.g. ticks and chorea).

3rd Mistake: Failing to differentiate the most common types of tremor.

1. Common causes of physiological tremor (Table 7.9).
2. Differentiating Tremor from Other Movement Disorders (Table 7.10).
3. Pathological Causes of Tremor in Older Children.

   Many diseases associated with tremor can be diagnosed by observing the tremor itself (Table 7.11).

TABLE 7.9 Common causes of physiological tremor

- Neonatal jitteriness, equivalent to tremor, (See Section Epilepsy) is very common, and needs to be differentiated from seizure caused by hypoglycaemia or hypocalcaemia. Normal jitteriness has no abnormal gaze or eye movement

- Infants of diabetic mothers are frequently jittery even with normal blood glucose and calcium

- Neonatal jitteriness typically can be provoked by stimulation of the baby or by stretching a joint. There is no decrease in oxygen saturation, no associated bradycardia or tachycardia, or increase in blood pressure. EEG record is normal

- Physiological tremor probably occurs in most individuals when the arms are at rest or when extended. Amplitude is barely visible with naked eyes. Frequency is <6 Hz before the age of 9 years. This is enhanced by anxiety, stress, cold exposure or caffeine intake. More subtle tremor can be demonstrated by holding a piece of paper on the outstretched hands. Tremor is absent during sleep

TABLE 7.10 The main non-tremor movement disorders

Ticks	• Tics are sudden brief, jerks, non-rhythmic, intermittent and aimless motor movements or vocalisation that persist for at least 1 year. Movements include eye blinking, head jerking, sniffing and/or eye blinking that occur in an inappropriate context. Typical age of occurrence: 5–7 years
	• There is typical variability in severity with waxing and waning. Typically there is ability to suppress tics temporarily but this suppression often leads to discomfort or urge to proceed with the movements.
	• Tourette syndrome is associated with multiple motor movements and vocalisation (e.g. obscene words, compulsive behaviour) that occur daily before the age of 18 years and persist for at least 1 year
Chorea	• Chorea is a hyperkinetic movement disorder characterised by involuntary brief, more rapid than tremor, jerky movements that affect predominately large random muscles particularly the face
	• Sydenham's chorea is the best known type of chorea, which is one of the major criteria of rheumatic fever. It occurs months after group A-beta haemolytic streptococcal pharyngitis
Dystonia	• Is characterised by sustained or intermittent muscle contractures causing patterned often repetitive movements and twisting that worsens by voluntary action
	• Causes include cerebral palsy and drug-induced, e.g. neuroleptics, haloperidol
Athetosis	• Athetosis is characterised by slow writhing, non-rhythmic or stereotyped involuntary movements, typically affecting hands, feet and neck
	• Typically, the same regions of the body are repeatedly involved, unlike chorea
	• Classical example is athetotic cerebral palsy occurring antenatally by injuring the basal ganglia

(continued)

TABLE 7.10 (continued)

Myoclonia	• Myoclonus is characterised by sudden, shock-like, brief, non-rhythmic involuntary jerks that commonly occur physiologically at sleep onset • Myoclonus may occur as part of juvenile myoclonic epilepsy, neurodegenerative and mitochondrial diseases

TABLE 7.11 The main four types of tremor

Types	Characteristics	Example
Rest	Fine tremor, normal neurology, with muscular rigidity, bradykinesia	Physiological Psychogenic Juvenile Parkinson's disease
Postural	Bilateral, symmetric involving hands/arms	Essential tremor
Kinetic	Occurring during voluntary movement	Physiological, psychogenic
Intention	Associated ataxia, dysarthria	Cerebellar diseases

Essential Tremor (ET)

- ET is a chronic, slowly progressive neurological disorder that manifests as bilateral postural and kinetic tremor of the hands and arms, inherited as autosomal dominant.
- It involves the hands, arms and often affects the head, face and vocal cords.
- There is absence of other neurological signs, so ET is a diagnosis of exclusion.
- Tremor occurs during voluntary movement such as writing and becomes obvious during spiral and line drawing, and pouring water from one cup to another.

Drug-Induced Tremor

- Drug addiction (e.g. cocaine, heroin, amphetamine) among pregnant women has increased steadily over years. The result is increased incidence of neonatal withdrawal syndrome with irritability, jitteriness and occasionally seizures. Obtaining a detailed maternal drug history is essential.

- Tremor may be caused by several medications, including asthma medications (e.g. β-2 agonists, theophylline), anticonvulsants (e.g. valproaite), and tricyclic antidepressants. Although tremor by β-2 agonist is benign, parents should be aware of this adverse effects when the medication is prescribed.

Metabolic Tremor

- In any child with progressive or acute tremor, serious conditions such as Wilson's disease, hyperthyroidism, hypoglycaemia, hypocalcaemia, neuroblastoma and pheochromocytoma must be excluded.
- Diagnosis of Wilson's disease is by ceruloplasmin and copper in serum and urine.

Psychogenic Tremor

- This type of tremor has a bizarre, asymmetric and abrupt-onset, with inconsistent non-symmetric movement, and spontaneous remission.
- Typically the tremor increases with attention and decreases with distractibility.
- It is a diagnosis of exclusion of other types of tremor.

Juvenile Parkinson's Disease (JPD)

- JPD is a rare movement disorder caused by degeneration of the basal ganglia leading to a loss of the neurotransmitter dopamine and pigmented neurone loss in the substantia nigra.
- The inherited autosomal recessive form of JPD is distinguished from the more prevalent idiopathic form by its early onset age, slower disease progress, occasional associated dystonia, and long-lasting response to low doses of L-dopa.
- Like in adults, JPD is characterised clinically by resting tremor, bradykinesia, rigidity and postural instability.

7.6   Large Head

Introduction/Core Messages
- Large and misshapen head is a very common reason for referral to paediatrician or paediatric surgeon.
- The measurement of the head circumference (HC) is a direct reflection of the brain volume, is a marker for development during the gestation and the first few years of life, and is useful in screening for abnormal head.
- The main two important entities of increased HC (> 2 standard deviations=SD) are macrocephaly (intracranial contents) and megalencephaly (oversize and overweight brain parenchyma).

Differential Diagnosis
Macrocephaly
Megalencephaly
Increased intracranial pressure
Hydrocephalus
Metabolic/storage diseases
Cerebral gigantism
Achondroplasia

Misdiagnosis is due to:
  1st mistake: lack of definition of large head.
  2nd mistake: failing to differentiate various main causes of large head.

1. Diagnostic Criteria of a Large Head

- Large head is defined as a head circumference (HC) greater than 2 standard deviations (i.e. greater than 98% centile on growth chart) above the mean for age, sex and duration of gestation.
- An enlarged head size with an occipito-frontal circumference of ≥2 SD is either due to intracranial contents including bone (macrocephaly) or overgrowth of the cerebrum

(megalencephaly). Differentiating between these two groups is essential because they represent differential disorders with different diagnostic approach, prognosis and treatment.

2. Main Causes of Large Head
    Macrocephaly (HC > 2 SD)

- This type of large head is due to non-parenchymal intracranial anomalies, e.g. bone skull structure, enlargement of the subarachnoid space, hydrocephalus, subdural haematoma, AV malformation and increased intracranial pressure.
- Macrocephaly is commonly inherited as autosomal dominant (familial macrocephaly) in over 50% of cases. It is more common in boys who inherit the condition from the parents, more often from their fathers. Therefore measurement of HC of the parents is essential. The condition is usually benign and children are developmentally normal.
- Children with macrocephaly and enlarging HC may be victims of child abuse (such as shaken baby syndrome) causing subdural haematoma. An important diagnostic clue is retinal haemorrhage.

Megalencephaly (Increased HC ≥ 2 SD due to brain growth)

- Megalencephaly is an increased growth of cerebral parenchyma (oversized and overweight brain) that presents either at birth or acquired postnatally. It occurs more frequently in children with developmental disability, e.g. children with autism spectrum disorder (ASD) are associated with megalencephaly in >90% of cases.
- Megalencephaly is divided into 3 main categories:

    - Idiopathic: familial benign.
    - Metabolic: e.g. defects of organic acids, leukodystrophy, lysosomal storage disease.
    - Anatomical: e.g. Achondroplasia, Sotos syndrome, neurofibromatosis.

Increased Intracranial Pressure = ICP (see also Sect. 7.3 Headache)

- ICP is characterised by a HC measurement that is crossing the centile line upwards, together with features of ICP.
- ICP in infants is characterised by irritability, poor feeding, vomiting and high-pitched cry. Late signs: tense or full fontanelle, sutures widely separated with prominent skull veins and downward gaze of the eyes (these presentations are nowadays unusual).
- Older children present with headache, vomiting, visual defects, changes of personality and behaviour.

Plagiocephaly

- This common condition is usually caused by preferential sleeping position and is characterised by flattening of one side or the whole of the baby's occiput. It is usually not associated with large HC but can be mistaken as such.
- The greatest deformity usually occurs in the first 3 months. The incidence has increased dramatically because of "Back to Sleep" campaign to reduce the incidence of sudden infant death syndrome.
- It is more common in premature infants, infants with hypotonicity and in those with developmental delay.
- Its importance is entirely cosmetic, and the shape of the head will usually correct itself by 12–18 months.
- The diagnosis of plagiocephaly is clinical and a skull X-ray to confirm the patency of the skull sutures is usually unnecessary.
- Characteristic signs (best detected when standing behind the infant and looking from above) include:
  - The head flattening is associated with compensatory ipsilateral protrusion or bulge of the forehead.
  - Elevation of the ipsilateral orbit and eyebrow.
  - Anteriorly positioned ipsilateral ear.
  - Normal separation of the skull sutures with no palpable bony ridges.

Further Reading

El-Radhi AS, et al. Essential paediatric in primary care: Radcliffe; 2014.

Uldall P, Alving J, Hansen LK, et al. A misdiagnosis of epilepsy in children admitted to a tertiary centre with paroxysmal events. Arch Dis Child. 2006;91(3):219–21.

Ungar A, Ceccofiglio A, Pescini F, et al. Epilepsy coexist in possible and drug-resistant epilepsy overlap between epilepsy and syncope study (OESYS). BMC Neurol. 2017;17:45.

Okubo Y, Matsuura M, Asai K, et al. Epileptiform EEG discharges in healthy children: prevalence, emotional and behavioural correlates, and genetic influences. Epilepsia. 1994;35(4):832–41.

Seneviratne U, Cook MJ, D'Souza WJ. Electroencephalography in the diagnosis of genetic generalized epilepsy syndromes. Front Neurol. 2017;8:499.

Louis ED, Kuo SH, Tate WH, et al. Cerebellar pathology in childhood-onset vs. adult-onset essential tremor. Neurosci Lett. 2017;659:69–74.

Chapter 8
Bone and Joint

8.1 Arthritis

Introduction/Core Messages
- A detailed discussion on arthritis, which compromises more than 100 different diseases, is beyond the scope of this book. In short, arthritis may be monoarthritis, oligoarthritis (<5 joints) or polyarthritis (5 or more joints).
- When a child presents with arthritis, the first question: is it monoarthritis, oligoarthritis or polyarthritis? That alone can restrict the differential diagnosis.
- Causes of polyarthritis include juvenile idiopathic arthritis (JIA), rheumatic fever (RF) and vasculitis. The main causes of oligoarthritis are trauma, septic arthritis, juvenile idiopathic arthritis (JIA), reactive arthritis (ReA), Lyme disease, transient synovitis, neoplastic and TB arthritis.
- JIA and ReA are forms of autoimmune arthritis; the latter develops 1–3 weeks an infection (viral or intes-

tinal infection, e.g. Campylobacter, Salmonella or Yersinia).
- JIA is the most important type of arthritis, and is classified into systemic-onset (associated with high remittent fever, rash, generalised lymphadenopathy, hepatosplenomegaly, serositis), oligoarthritis and polyarthritis.

Differential Diagnosis

Common	Rare
Juvenile idiopathic arthritis	Rheumatic fever
Reactive arthritis	Arthritis of IBD
Transient synovitis	Lyme disease
Septic arthritis	Neoplastic arthritis
Collagen	TB arthritis
Vasculitis	

Misdiagnosis is due to:

1st mistake: Failing to establish the diagnosis of JIA as the most important arthritis in childhood.

2nd mistake: Failing to differentiate other important causes of polyarthritis.

3rd mistake: Failing to establish the diagnoses of common oligo- and monoarthritis.

1. Diagnostic Features of JIA

- JIA is a heterogeneous group of arthritis of unknown aetiologies that compromises several disease categories mainly systemic arthritis, polyarthritis and oligoarthritis (Table 8.1).
- JIA is characterised by arthritis of more than 6 weeks' duration, presenting <16 years of age (mean age 4 years) and unexplained by known causes. It is a diagnosis of exclusion other possible causes of arthritis.

TABLE 8.1 The three cardinal manifestations of JIA

- Systemic arthritis (10% of JIA) is characterised by arthritis (symmetric, polyarthritis) accompanied or preceded by:

  - Quotidian fever (daily occurring fever with one or two daily spikes) for at least two weeks' duration

  - Rash, generalised symmetrical lymphadenopathy, enlargement of the spleen or liver, and polyserositis (pleural or pericardial effusion or pericarditis)

  - The rash characteristically is fleeting, salmon-coloured, macular or maculopapular, occurring particularly when the temperature is elevated and subsides when fever settles. Males and females are equally affected

  - Other features include leukocytosis, anaemia, myocarditis and pericarditis

- The polyarticular onset or adult type (10–30% of JIA)

  - The onset is abrupt or insidious arthritis of several symmetrical large of small joints. Females are predominately affected; mean age 12 years

  - This group is divided into rheumatoid factor-positive and negative

  - Occasionally the patients present with systemic manifestations such as low grade fever, lymphadenopathy and recurrent rash

- Oligoarthritis or pauciarticular arthritis (50–80% of JIA) affecting predominately females younger than 6 years. The arthritis is typically asymmetric affecting mainly the knee joints. Uveitis and high ANA-level are common

---

- Uveitis may be the initial presentation of JIA, particularly with oligoarthritis. One third of children develop unilateral (even bilateral) loss of visual acuity. Regular eye checks are essential.
- Temporomandibular arthritis in JIA is a challenge joint to evaluate because of absence joint swelling. If untreated early, devastating effects occur on the form and function of it.

- FBC confirms leukocytosis, raised ESR, CRP and platelets
- Auto-antibodies (e.g. anti-nuclear antibodies) are positive in the majority of JIA
- Rheumatoid factor (RF) is rarely positive in JIA except in a small group with polyarthritis. If RF is positive it suggests a more aggressive disease with bone erosion compared to those with negative RF

2. Other Causes of Polyarthritis
Rheumatic Fever (RF)

- RF is characterised by migratory arthritis occurring 2–3 weeks following an untreated group A beta-haemolytic streptococcal pharyngitis.
- Diagnosis is established by Jones criteria (Table 8.2).
- These criteria were revised in 2015. Fever of 38.0°C has been accepted as minor criterion in the revised criteria instead of the previous level of 38.5°C. Monoarthritis has become a major criterion along with polyarthritis and an ESR of 30 mm/h instead of previous 60 mm/h.

Polyarthritis due to Vasculitis

- Henoch–Schönlein Purpura (HSP) manifests with a rash of typical distribution (buttocks, external areas of elbows and knee joints) , abdominal pain and nephritis.
- Kawasaki disease (KD) is established by the criteria shown in the Table 8.3.

3. Oligoarthritis (4 or Fewer Joints Including Monoarthritis)
Septic Arthritis (SA)

- SA is defined as positive joint fluid culture for bacteria and/or WBC count in the joint fluid of >50,000 cells/mm (predominately polymorphonuclear cells) with or without positive blood culture (positive in about 50%).
- SA is almost always monoarticular involving predominately large joints. Children with immunocompromised status or haemoglobinopathy are at high risk of developing SA.

TABLE 8.2 Accepted Jones criteria of RF as revised in 2015

Manifestation	Presentation
Major	
Carditis (pan-carditis, subclinical carditis, valvulitis)	Tachycardia, gallop rhythm, cardiomegaly Cardiac failure
Polyarthritis/monoarthritis/arthralgia	Migratory polyarthritis
Chorea (rare)	Present with abrupt aimless movement
Erythema marginatum	Transient erythematous rash over the trunk
Subcutaneous nodules	Non-tender, nodules on the joints
Minor	
Fever 38.0 °C, arthralgia, grade 1 heart block, (ECG), ESR $\geq$30; CRP $\geq$3.0	
(In addition to: Supporting evidence of recent streptococcal infection)	

TABLE 8.3 Diagnostic criteria of Kawasaki disease

Fever persisting for at least 5 days plus at least four of the following five:

1. bilateral, painless conjunctival inflammation without exudates

2. changes of the oropharynx mucosa, cracking lips, strawberry tongue

3. acute unilateral non-purulent cervical lymphadenopathy >1.5 cm

4. polymorphous rash, primarily truncal

5. changes of peripheral extremities: oedema and/or erythema of hands and feet

- Clinically, SA manifests as severe joint pain with restricted joint mobility, high fever >39.5°C, in addition of signs of arthritis.
- Joint aspiration is diagnostic (see the definition above). FBC shows leukocytosis with high CRP/ESR. Ultrasound scan and joint x-ray show may show periosteal reaction. Bone scan is often positive.

Juvenile Idiopathic Arthritis presenting as mono-or oligoarthritis (see above JIA)

Reactive Arthritis (ReA)

It is an autoimmune arthritis that develops in response to an infection elsewhere in the body, most commonly a viral URT or intestinal infection (Campylobacter, Salmonella, Shigella or Yersinia). ReA is one of the most common causes of arthritis. Characteristic features include:

- History of infection occurring 1–3 weeks prior to the onset of arthritis.
- Arthritis occurring in weight-bearing joints (knee and ankle).
- Commonly associated with the human leukocyte antigen HLA-B27.
- Joint aspirate showing an increased WBC but is sterile to culture.
- Post-streptococcal ReA differs from RF in the absence of heart, CNS and skin lesions in addition to poor response to aspirin.

Lyme Disease (LD)

- Following a tick bite, patient develops flu-like illness with a characteristic annular skin rash (erythema migrans), which develops at the site of the tick bite. Antibiotics at this stage may prevent subsequent stages.
- The second stage follows 2–12 weeks after the tick bite and is characterised by disseminated infection causing aseptic meningitis and cranial neuritis (most commonly

presenting as facial palsy) and carditis (most commonly presenting as atrioventricular block or myocarditis).

- The third stage is characterised by intermittent or persistent arthritis affecting particularly the knees, shoulders and ankles. Involvement of small joints of hands and feet are uncommon. Migratory arthralgia may occur during early stage of LD.
- Diagnosis is established by clinical features, travelling or living in an endemic area, and positive IgG, IgM, PCR. CSF often detects lymphocytic pleocytosis and high protein.

Transient Synovitis (TS)

- The diagnosis of TS is made when a generally health-looking child presents with limping but still walking, with low-grade or no fever, and a history of a viral upper respiratory tract infection. One hip is usually affected.
- Investigation such as blood WBC, CRP and ESR are usually normal. Joint aspiration is generally not required, but if it is performed it shows a WBC count of <50,000/mm in the joint fluid. Hip ultrasound scan often shows increased fluid in the joint.
- TS is a self-limited arthritis, usually lasting 1–3 weeks.

Neoplastic Arthritis (e.g. leukaemia, lymphoma) is uncommon. Diagnostic clues:

- Patients with rheumatic diseases such as JIA or SLE are at increased risk of developing some forms of malignancies, e.g. haematological cancers or lymphoma. The disease and the use of immune-suppressants predispose to this development.
- The initial presentation of leukaemia or lymphoma often consists of arthralgia and arthritis that typically causes limb pain, often nocturnal, in association with weight loss, hepatomegaly, anaemia and thrombocytopenia. Blast cells in the peripheral blood smear are often present.

TB Arthritis

- Tuberculous osteoarthritis is a rare form of extra-pulmonary TB (about 1% among all children with TB). The increased incidence in recent years is due to associated immunodeficiency diseases (such as HIV) or the use of immunosuppressant drugs to treat arthritic conditions such as JIA.
- The onset of TB-arthritis is typically insidious with local symptoms of pain, tenderness and limitation of movements. Other symptoms are related specifically to TB including, malaise, weight loss, fatigue, low-grade-fever, peaking at night with night sweating.
- Diagnosis is made by positive Mantoux test, interferon-gamma release assay (the currently preferred test), synovial biopsy and MRI, which the image of choice.

Further Reading

Barut K, Androvic A, Sahin S, et al. Juvenile idiopathic arthritis. Balkan Med J. 2017;34(2):90–101.

Chapter 9
Urology

9.1 Bedwetting (Nocturnal Enuresis)

Introduction/Core Messages

- Bedwetting (Nocturnal enuresis) presents either in isolation (monosymptomatic NE) or in association with UTI, vulvovaginitis, daytime incontinence, urge, hesitancy, straining symptoms of urination, post-void dribbling or dysfunctional voiding (non-monosymptomatic NE).
- NE is divided into primary nocturnal enuresis (PNE) (continue to wet beyond the age of 5 years), affecting 80% of children, and secondary nocturnal enuresis (SNE) (restarting bedwetting after a previous dry period >6 months) in 20% of children.
- Causes of PNE include genetic (on chromosome 12 and 13), delayed maturation, sleep disorders and antidiuretic hormone (ADH) deficiency. Causes of SNE include urinary tract infection (UTI), emotional stress, type 1 diabetes (T1D), child abuse, diabetes insipidus (DI), obstructive sleep apnoea (OSA) and seizure.

© Springer Nature Switzerland AG 2021   175
A. S. El-Radhi, *Avoiding Misdiagnosis in Pediatric Practice*,
In Clinical Practice, https://doi.org/10.1007/978-3-030-41750-5_9

Differential Diagnosis of Underlying Causes

Common	Rare
Primary nocturnal enuresis (mostly genetic)	Renal tubular acidosis
Secondary nocturnal enuresis (SNE)	Sickle cell anaemia
Compulsive fluid drinking	Bladder neck obstruction
Type 1 diabetes (T1D)	Diabetes insipidus
Developmental delay	Chronic renal failure

Misdiagnosis is *due* to:

1. Mistake: Failing to differentiate between monosymptomatic and complicated NE.
2. Mistake: Failing to recognise other underlying causes of nocturnal enuresis.

1. Differentiating Monosymptomatic NE from Non-monosymptomatic NE.

    Table 9.1 shows diagnostic criteria of mono-symptomatic NE: The following disorders are associated with non-monosymptomatic NE:

    Urinary tract infection (UTI) is confirmed by urine culture and defined as a single growth of bacteria of >100,000 colony-forming unit per mL, and combination of clinical features presenting as an:

    - Upper UTI is defined as UTI with a fever of 38 °C or higher, usually without a source of infection. This is the most common presentation of UTI in infancy.
    - Lower UTI is defined as a collection of well-recognised symptoms including dysuria, frequency, incontinence and supra-pubic pain in toilet-trained children.

    Urinary incontinence (UI) is a common problem often associated with frequent urination, urge symptom and nocturnal enuresis (NE). It indicates involuntary loss of urine during the daytime (diurnal) after the age of 5 years.

    Painful or burning urination during or immediately after urination, termed dysuria, is often accompanied by other urinary symptoms such as frequency, urgency or hesitancy.

TABLE 9.1 Diagnostic criteria of monosymptomatic NE

- NE is defined as the involuntary voiding of urine during sleep at least three times a week for at least three months in a child 5 years or older. It is the most common chronic urinary childhood complaint affecting 10% of children aged 5 years, 5% aged 10 years and 1–2% at pubertal age.

- Normal physical examination, including lumbosacral area and lower limbs.

- Absence of UTI, diurnal incontinence, glycosuria, signs of renal tubular acidosis.

Frequent urination, the term indicates frequent (more than seven a day in school-age children) voids of small amounts of urine, often associated with urgency.

Vulvovaginitis, usually non-specific, may occur in up to 70% of girls, which is caused by poor perineal hygiene, tendency of the labia minora to open on squatting, and close proximity of the anal orifice to the vagina allowing transfer of bacteria to the vulva, urethra and bladder. Other contributory factors include the use of antibiotics and steroids, wearing tight knickers and tights, and the use of irritants such as detergents and bubble bath.

Dysfunctional Voiding (DV)

- DV applies to children who habitually contract bladder detrusor muscle against closed urethral sphincter during voiding. DV is usually associated with constipation, painful local irritation (e.g. vulvovaginitis, balanitis), fear of unclean toilet and urge symptom of urination with attempt to avoid voiding.

- Persistent dysfunctional voiding may lead to non-neurogenic neurogenic bladder, which is characterised by failure of the external sphincter to relax during voiding leading to trabeculated bladder, hydronephrosis and renal failure.

2. Other Causes of NE (see Section of Polyuria)
   Compulsive Drinking (Primary Polydipsia)

- Young children with compulsive drinking are easily recognised by the long history, absence of weight loss or failure to thrive. Serum osmolality is 300–800 m0sm/kg

upon thirst. A urine osmolality >600 m0sm/kg during the water deprivation test supports the diagnosis.
- Children with compulsive drinking are usually pre-school aged, healthy and thriving. In older children, the condition is frequently associated with psychiatric disorders, and hyponatraemia and water intoxication are commonly observed. Compulsive drinking needs to be differentiated from DI (see below).

Diabetes Type 1 (TID)

- Childhood presentation of T1D is usually with characteristic features including polyuria symptoms of polyuria, polydipsia, weight loss and high blood glucose. The goals of treatment are near normalisation of glucose metabolism (HbA1c < 7.5% = 58.5 mmol).
- Diagnosis is established by high blood glucose (HbA1c $\geq$ 6.5% or fasting BG: 7.0 mmol = 126 mg/dL). Urinalysis will confirm glycosuria and ketones in T1D.

Diabetes Insipidus (DI)

- DI is characterised by a triad: polyuria (urine output of 4ml/kg/h or >50ml/kg/day), polydipsia (>2L/m^2/day) and failure to thrive. Other symptoms include seizures and fever of unknown origin. The diagnosis of DI rests on high plasma osmolality and low urine osmolality. The differential diagnosis between DI and compulsive drinking is discussed above.
- In children, nephrogenic DI (mainly X-linked, is more common in children, and is caused by renal tubular unresponsiveness to vasopressin) than central DI (autosomal recessive or dominant inheritance, and is caused defective vasopressin action). MRI of the pituitary may show an absence of a bright signal that is considered to be pathognomonic for this type of DI.
- Diagnostic for DI during water deprivation test (WDT): serum osmolality >300 mOsm/kg and a urine osmolality <300 mOsm/kg. Plasma copeptin (a peptide from posterior pituitary) levels may replace in the future the WDT as the gold standard test.

Renal Tubular Acidosis

- The fourth most important cause of polyuria is renal tubular acidosis. Children may present with dehydration, failure to thrive, anorexia and vomiting.
- Diagnosis is by finding glycosuria, low serum bicarbonate and potassium, and hyperchloraemia.

9.2   Blood in Urine (Haematuria)

Introduction/Core Messages
- When a child presents with blood in urine, doctors should determine that it is actually haematuria.
- Proteinuria in association with haematuria is very suggestive of renal origin of the haematuria. Casts, particularly RBCs casts, indicate a diagnosis of glomerulonephritis.
- Gross haematuria indicates that blood is seen with naked eyes. Microscopic haematuria is more common (incidence 1–2% of school-age children) and is defined as >5 RBC/HPF in the urine sediment of centrifuged freshly voided urine.
- In contrast to gross haematuria, the majority of patients (70-80%) with micro-haematuria have no clinically identifiable cause for the haematuria. Isolated microscopic haematuria is common in healthy children and is often transient. Persistent microscopic haematuria indicates >5RBCs per high power field at monthly intervals, and it requires investigation to exclude serious causes of haematuria.
- The haematuria of glomerular disease is usually uniformly red, without clots or pain. An exception is Henoch–Schönlein purpura (HSP), which is associated with abdominal pain.
- Causes of painful non-glomerular haematuria include urolithiasis, trauma or lower urinary tract infection (UTI).

Differential Diagnosis

Common	Rare
Anti-streptococcal glomerulonephritis (PSGN)	Coagulopathies
IgA nephropathy	Renal tumour
Hypercalciuria	Obstructive uropathy
Henoch-Schönlein-Purpura (HSP)	Renal artery/vein thrombosis
Renal stones	Systemic lupus erythematosus (SLE)
Drugs	Benign familial haematuria
Urinary tract infection (UTI)	Alport syndrome
	Goodpasture syndrome (with pulmonary haemorrhage)
	Haemorrhagic cystitis (following Cyclophosphamide)
	Polycystic kidney disease
	Vascular (e.g. renal vein thrombosis)
	Haemolytic–uraemic syndrome (HUS)
	Alport syndrome
	Polycystic kidneys

Misdiagnosis is due to:

1. Mistake: Failing to differentiate blood from other blood-appearing substances in the urine.
2. Mistake: Failing to recognise pathologies causing blood in urine in neonates.
3. Mistakes: Failing to recognise common pathologies causing haematuria in older children.
1. Urinary Substances Appearing as Blood

- Characteristics of blood are shown in Table 9.2.

- Neonatal vaginal discharge due to maternal hormonal withdrawal is often mistaken for haematuria particularly when the blood is mixed with urine. Parents should be reassured.
- The presence of red-brown or pink discolouration on the nappies occurring during the first few days of life is often urate crystals that can easily be mistaken as blood. This is a benign condition and improves rapidly with increased fluid intake.
- Intense exercise can cause rhabdomyolysis and red urine.
- Red urine may be due to drugs (e.g. rifampicin, nitrofurantoin), metabolic (e.g. porphyrins, methaemoglobin), pigments (e.g. haemoglobin, myoglobin) and food (e.g. beets, blackberries). The red colour after ingestion of beetroots is due to unmetabolised betalain pigments.
- In these conditions, urinalysis will be negative for red blood cells. Methaemoglobin can be measured by co-oximeter.

2. Haematuria in Neonates.

   Red staining of the nappy can be due to either true blood with RBCs or urates. Urinalysis should be performed to differentiate between the two.

   Haemorrhagic Disease of the Newborn (HDN).

- Although the most common manifestation of HDN is melena, babies may present with haematuria.

TABLE 9.2 Characteristics of blood

• Blood is composed of blood cells (45%) suspended in plasma (55%)
• Blood has five main functions: delivering oxygen and nutrients, removing metabolic products waste, forming blood clots, carrying cells and antibodies and regulating body temperature
• Confirmation of blood is by laboratory finding of red blood cells (RBCs)

- HDN occurs in 1 in 200–400 neonates who did not receive vitamin K prophylaxis. Vit K, 1.0 mg IV.

Urinary Tract Infection (UTI)

- Neonatal UTI is usually associated with nonspecific symptoms and signs of septicaemia including ill-looking appearance, poor feeding and weight gain, poor body temperature control and jaundice.
- UTI affects usually male newborns caused by haematogenous bacterial spread to the kidney.
- Positive urine and blood cultures, and high inflammatory markers confirm the diagnosis.

Nephrocalcinosis

- Nephrocalcinosis is not uncommon in premature babies and it can be seen in up to 40%. Risk factors include the use of loop diuretics, prematurity, metabolic acidosis and renal tubular acidosis. It predisposes to UTI and haematuria. Resolution occurs in the majority of cases.
- Diagnosis is established by renal ultrasonography.

Neonatal Renal Vein and Artery Thrombosis

- Common presentation of neonatal renal vein and artery thrombosis is gross haematuria, thrombocytopenia and abdominal mass (in vein thrombosis). Hypertension occurs with arterial thrombosis, and this sign should be searched for by repeated blood pressure measurements.
- Diagnosis is made by renal ultrasonography and selective renal venography or arteriography.

3. Haematuria in Older Children
   Post-Streptococcal Glomerulonephritis (PSGN)

   - In PSGN, the most common cause of gross haematuria worldwide, the urine is uniformly red, either brownish-red or dark brown (Coca-Cola colour), not pink-tinged. Significant abdominal pain is usually absent, except cases with HSP.

- The presence of proteinuria with haematuria and casts, particularly RBCs casts, indicates a diagnosis of glomerulonephritis. Throat swab for streptococci group A and ASO-titre will establish PSGN.
- Gross haematuria in association with mild oedema, hypertension and high creatinine suggests nephritic syndrome, while gross oedema and proteinuria suggest nephrotic syndrome.

IgA Nephropathy

- IgA nephropathy is the most common cause of glomerulonephritis in Western World and the most common cause of recurrent painless haematuria affecting typically children aged 8–10 years. Haematuria often subsides but soon to be followed by microscopic haematuria. There is usually initial mild proteinuria (<0.5 g/day).
- IgA nephropathy may present as progressive kidney disease and end-stage renal failure with hypertension.
- Gross haematuria following an URTI suggests IgA nephropathy. Diagnosis is by renal biopsy showing glomerular IgA immune deposits (not established by serum complement or IGA levels).

Urinary Tract Infection

- It is wrong to make a diagnosis of UTI based on urine RBCs or protein or both. Positive nitrite and WBCs in the dipstick are more important indicators in suggesting UTI than these 2 indices protein and/or RBCs.
- UTI is defined as a single growth of bacteria of >100,000 colony-forming unit per mL, and combination of clinical features presenting as an:
- Upper UTI defined as UTI with a fever of 38 °C or higher, usually without a source of infection. This is the most common presentation of UTI in infancy. Lower UTI is associated with afebrile symptoms including dysuria, frequency, incontinence and supra-pubic pain.

Renal Stones

- Haematuria in association with abdominal pain suggests UTI, HSP, renal stone or tumour. An urgent urinalysis is required.
- While adults and older children (>7 to 8 years of age) with urolithiasis present nearly always with severe flank pain, colic and haematuria, younger children usually present with diffuse abdominal pain, UTI, micro-haematuria, or remain asymptomatic for years.

- Renal ultrasound scan has a high specificity >90% and lower sensitivity. Metabolic evaluation (calcium or non-calcium stones) is required. Plain abdominal X-ray is no longer used.

Henoch–Schönlein Purpura (HSP)

- HSP (or IgA vasculitis as the new term) is the most common vasculitis in children with IgA immune deposits affecting small blood vessels. Renal involvement occurs in 20–40% of cases, determining long-term prognosis.
- Diagnosis is clinical with the following features: abdominal pain, arthritis, typical purpuric skin rash affecting the legs and buttocks in addition to nephritis occurring in 20-40% of cases.

Metabolic   Causes   of   Haematuria   (See   also Hypercalciuria in 9.3)

- Microscopic haematuria is common in children and is often idiopathic. The most known cause of microscopic haematuria without proteinuria is hypercalciuria (about 25% of cases), and is confirmed by urinary calcium/creatinine ratio and elevated calcium excretion of >4 mg/kg in 24 h urine collection. Hypercalcaemic hypercalciuria (e.g. hyperparathyroidism) is confirmed by high serum calcium.
- Other metabolic causes include cystinuria, hyperoxaluria and renal tubular acidosis.

Renal Tumour (Nephroblastoma = Wilms)

- Nephroblastoma is the most common urological malignancy in children. The tumour commonly presents as a unilateral (5–10% are bilateral) abdominal mass in a young child (median age 3 years), often detected by a parent (in over 80% of cases). Other presentations include fever (reported incidence 23–50% of cases), haematuria and hypertension (caused by rennin secretion). Cough and dyspnoea may occur due to pulmonary metastasis.
- Diagnosis is established by renal ultrasonography and CT scan.

Schistosomiasis

- In many countries, e.g. Egypt, haematuria is mostly due to a prevalent parasitic infection, Schistosoma haematobium. Other symptoms include frequent and painful urination. The infection is complicated by mega-ureter, hydronephrosis and calcified bladder.
- Diagnosis is made by detection of eggs in urine and faeces, or biopsy of the bladder. Eosinophilia is common.

9.3   Frequent Urination

Introduction/Core Messages
- Frequent urination is a common symptom with usual underlying causes in children. The condition can impact children physically, socially and psychologically. Therefore early diagnosis and treatment are essential to prevent adverse effects on kidney and bladder function as well restoring psychosocial well-being.
- In paediatrics, the most common cause of frequent urination is an overactive bladder with or without UTI. The condition has to be differentiated from polyuria (frequent of large amount of urine), and incontinence (involuntary loss of urine). Female children are more affected than males.

Differential Diagnosis

Common	Rare
Lower urinary tract infection (UTI)	Urethritis (e.g. Reiter's syndrome)
Vulvovaginitis	Ectopic ureter
Overactive bladder (detrusor instability)	Vaginal voiding
Diuretics	Bladder outlet obstruction
Pollakiuria and anxiety (Daytime frequent urination)	Congenital stricture of the urethra
Developmental delay (incl. neurogenic bladder)	

Misdiagnosis is due to:

1. Mistake: Failing to establish characteristics of frequent urination.
2. Mistake: Failing to differentiate frequent intermittent urination from continuous urination.
3. Mistake: Failing to differentiate frequent urination from polyuria.
4. Mistake: Failing to establish other causes of frequent urination.

1. Characteristics of Frequent Urination
    Diagnostic considerations of frequent urination are shown in Table 9.3.

2. Differentiating Frequent from Continuous Urination.
    Frequent voiding may be due to continuous incontinence due to posterior urethral valve obstruction in boys, and ectopic ureter in girls. Diagnostic criteria of both conditions are shown in Table 9.4.

TABLE 9.3 Clinical Features of Frequent Urination

- The term indicates frequent (more than seven a day in school-age children) voids of small amounts of urine, often associated with urgency. In infancy, voiding is physiologically frequent, as often as 15–20 times a day, occurring by reflex bladder contraction mediated by sympathetic nerve system (T10-L2) and parasympathetic nerve system (S2-S4).

- In older children, bladder control is achieved through gradual bladder enlargement, leading to an increase of bladder capacity, cortical inhibition of the reflex bladder contraction, and the ability to tighten the external sphincter to prevent incontinence.

- The most common cause of frequent urination is overactive bladder that is associated with uninhibited detrusor contraction during the storage phase of bladder function.

- Pollakiuria (from the Greek word "pollakis" meaning many times) is the second most common cause of frequent urination that occurs as a result of stress-related problems, but without dysuria or systemic disease. There is sudden onset of frequent voiding every 5–10 min, in a previously toilet-trained child. It often disappears suddenly in 2–3 months. Typical age of occurrence is 4–8 years.

- Dysfunctional voiding occurs in children who habitually contract the urethral sphincter or pelvic floor during voiding causing obstruction. Children do not take time to empty their bladder so that they can hurry back to play.

- Diagnosis begins with keeping, for at least three consecutive days, a voiding diary that contains data on the hours and volumes of voided urine to establish the frequency and functional bladder capacity.

TABLE 9.4 Diagnostic criteria of posterior urethral valve and ectopic ureter

- Posterior urethral valve is one of the most common causes of bladder outlet obstruction in male children. Diagnosis can be made by antenatal ultrasound scan and established by voiding cystourethrography showing dilated posterior valve and a narrow urethra, bladder neck hypertrophy and trabeculation.

- Ectopic ureter is any ureter, single or duplex, that does not open in the usual trigonal region of the bladder (e.g. uterus, vagina or perineum). Over 80% of cases are associated with duplex system. Presentation is persistent dribbling incontinence. Diagnosis is established by ultrasonography and CT scan urography showing duplex kidney and the route of the ectopic ureter.

3. Differentiating Frequent Urination from Polyuria

- In the differential diagnosis of frequent urination, the most important aspect is to exclude polyuria. Mothers are usually good historian. Observing the child's urination helps establish the diagnosis.
- Arrange a urine collection over 12 or 24 h to establish the diagnosis if necessary (see Section of Polyuria).

4. Other Causes of Frequent Urination
   Urinary Tract Infection (UTI)
   Diagnosis of UTI rests on certain diagnostic criteria (Table 9.5).
   Vulvovaginitis (see also Section of vaginal discharge)

- Non-specific vulvovaginitis is common in pre-pubertal girls, which is caused by poor perineal hygiene, tendency of the labia minora to open on squatting, and close proximity of the anal orifice to the vagina allowing transfer of faecal bacteria to the vagina.
- Other contributory factors include the use of systemic antibiotics and steroids, wearing tight-fitting clothes such as tight, and the use of irritants such as detergents and bubble bathing.

TABLE 9.5 Diagnostic criteria of UTI

- A febrile child without a focus of infection whose urine showed positive nitrite and leukocytes in the dipstick testing is very suggestive of having UTI. Negative result of these two indicators virtually excludes UTI. A positive urinalysis is defined as 5 or more WBC per high power field.

- Urine culture is the ultimate tool to confirm UTI, which is diagnosed if the urine shows a count of >100,000 colonies/ml of a single bacterial growth. Suprapubic puncture is important for accurate diagnosis during infancy, and a culture of 50,000 colonies is diagnostic. In older children mid-stream urine sample is sufficient.

- Laboratory tests: Leukocytosis >15,000 and high CRP >40mg/L support the diagnosis. CRP is particularly valuable when fever has been present >12 h. Procalcitonin (PCT) >0.5 ng/mL is a major predictor (compared to WBC count and CRP) for identifying children with acute upper urinary tract infection (pyelonephritis) during early stages of UTI.

- Children with vulvovaginitis present with pruritis, frequent urination, dysuria, enuresis, sleep disturbance or erythema of the vulva.

   Labial Adhesions

- Labial adhesions, defined as partly (involving the area between the posterior and midline of the labia minora, leaving a small gap anteriorly for passage of urine) or completely fused labia minora. It usually occurs in girls 1–2 years of age, and mostly caused by hypo-oestrogenic state. Prevalence is about 2%. The condition usually causes a great parental anxiety.

- Girls are often asymptomatic, or present with frequent or continuous passage of urine. Typically, passage of urine occurs during and after the girl stands up.

Hypercalciuria

- Hypercalciuria is a common metabolic disorder causing recurrent haematuria, renal stones, dysuria, frequent urination, proteinuria, recurrent UTI, abdominal and back pain. Hypercalciuria is the most common cause of microscopic haematuria (25% of causes).
- Hypercalciuria may be idiopathic, caused by diet (excess sodium inhibit renal tubular calcium absorption), proximal tubular dysfunction (e.g. Fanconi syndrome) or vitamin D excess/toxicity in association with hypercalcaemia.
- Hypercalciuria is defined by calcium excretion of >4mg/kg per day in 24 h urine collection.

Child Abuse

- There is a strong link between child abuse (sexual, emotional and physical) and urological symptoms, even years after the abuse has occurred. This link should be kept in mind when a child presents with urinary frequency, urgency symptoms.
- History and physical examination usually confirm the diagnosis.

9.4   Painful Urination (Dysuria)

Introduction/Core Messages
- Painful or burning urination during or immediately after urination, termed dysuria, is often accompanied by other urinary symptoms such as frequency, urgency or hesitancy.
- Although this can sometimes be a sign of UTI, it is more commonly caused by vulvovaginitis, balanitis or urethritis. The majority of causes of dysuria are self-limiting and identified by physical examination with urine or discharge cultures.

- Children sometimes express itching as dysuria, and this is commonly seen with worm infestation. Children who have persistent dysuria and with a normal examination and negative cultures are likely to have either dysfunctional void or hypercalciuria.
- History and physical examination will usually confirm the underlying cause and determine whether any test is necessary.

Differential Diagnosis

Common	Rare
UTI	Sexual transmitted diseases
Atopic dermatitis	Sexual abuse
Balanitis	Reiter's syndrome (urethritis, arthritis, red eyes)
Hypercalciuria	Lichen planus
Urethritis/cystitis	Herpes simplex infection (peri-urethral)
Chemical irritation	

Misdiagnosis is due to:

1st mistake: failing to recognise that dysuria can exist in infancy.

2nd mistake: failing to establish common underlying causes of painful urination.

1. Dysuria in Infancy

- Painful urination may occur due to urethritis (usually confined to anterior bulbar urethra) caused by infection, as idiopathic urethritis, hypercalciuria, or part of Reiter's syndrome (associated with conjunctivitis and polyarthritis). Nappy dermatitis is most common cause of dysuria in infancy.

- Typical manifestations include irritability and crying, particularly during urination, frequent and straining urination, and possible urethral discharge. Haematuria (usually microscopic) may be present.
- Cystourethroscopy may be used for urethral disorders. Bladder sonography is indicated for urolithiasis.

2. Dysuria in Older Children

- Urinary tract infection (UTI), usually lower UTI, is the most common cause of dysuria.
- Meatal stenosis, abnormal narrowing of the urethral opening (meatus), may be congenital or acquired, e.g. after circumcision. Condition is characterised by upward, deflected urine, dysuria, urgency, frequency and prolonged urination. A child with meatal stenosis requires urgent attention to avoid potential chronic incomplete bladder emptying with subsequent UTI and kidney damage.
- Vulval lichen sclerosis is a chronic dermatosis of unknown aetiology characterised by white patches or plagues affecting vulva and anus, and causing irritation, dysuria and urinary incontinence. In males it is known as balanitis xerotica obliterans.
- Vulvovaginitis (see Section: Vaginal discharge).
- Foreign body, such as piece of toilet paper, can be trapped in the vagina and causes discharge and dysuria. Careful area inspection is essential.
- Threadworms (pinworms). Pruritis caused by these helminthic infection can cause as dysuria. Threadworms which normally infest the perianal area but occasionally spread to the vagina.
- Pelvic inflammatory disease (PID) in females may present with dysuria and abdominal pain. Asymptomatic infections with either N. gonorrhoeae or chlamydia trachomatis may lead to development of PID, which has serious consequences if left untreated.
- Sexual transmitted diseases (STD). A urethral or vaginal discharge in an adolescent is likely caused by an infection with either N. gonorrhoeae or chlamydia trachomatis.

- Urolithiasis is either due to urethral stone or stasis of blood in the urethra.
- Herpes simplex virus can cause painful urethritis with subsequent urine retention with dilation of the urinary tract system. Careful examination is important as vesicles of this virus may be tiny and inapparent.
- Hypercalciuria. In patients with normal examination and negative cultures, dysuria (often associated with microscopic haematuria) can be caused by hypercalciuria. A 24-h urine collection is indicated.

9.5   Urinary Incontinence

Introduction/Core Messages
- Urinary incontinence (UI) is a common problem presenting at primary care services. It is usually associated with frequent urination, urge symptom (due to overactive bladder) and nocturnal enuresis (NE). Other co-morbidities include dysfunctional voiding (contraction of the urethral sphincter or pelvic floor during voiding), psychological and behavioural problems.
- Daytime UI and NE are commonly co-exist. However, daytime UI is more prevalent than NE in girls whereas NE is more prevalent than UI in boys.
- Primary UI is usually intermittent (more commonly) or continuous associated with anatomical and/or neurological organic causes: congenital malformation of the ureter, neurogenic bladder caused by spina bifida, sacral agenesis and acquired degenerative or neoplastic disease of the CNS.
- Secondary UI (onset of symptoms after an asymptomatic period of ≥6 months) is usually associated with stressful event, constipation, type-1diabetes (T1D) and child abuse. The main causes of UI are an overactive bladder leading to urinary urge, and holding urine until the last min by suppressing the need

to void, until incontinence happens. Around 20–40% of children with UI have behavioural problems including ADHD, anxiety and antisocial behaviour.

Differential Diagnosis

Common	Rare
Unstable bladder	Ectopic ureter
Congenital malformation	Bladder outlet obstruction
Lower UTI	Chronic renal failure
Neurogenic bladder	Sacral agenesis
Giggle incontinence	Meningomyelocele
Labial adhesions	Vulval reflux of urine
	Lipomeningocele

Misdiagnosis is due to:

1. Mistake: Failing to consider basic knowledge on urinary incontinence.
2. Mistake: Failing to establish important secondary causes of urinary incontinence.

1. Basic Knowledge of Urinary Incontinence
    Basic knowledge of urinary incontinence is shown in Table 9.6.

2. Underlying Causes of Urinary Incontinence

   - **Labial fusion** is common affecting about 3% of pre-pubertal girls. The labia minora fuse, usually distally, allowing a tiny opening proximally. The pocket behind the fused labia acts as a reservoir from which urine is leaking when the girl is standing or playing.
   - **Hinman syndrome** is a non-neurogenic (spine is normal) voiding dysfunction caused by uncoordinated activity of the detrusor muscle, bladder neck and

TABLE 9.6 Useful information of urinary incontinence in children

- Urinary incontinence is defined as unintentional leakage of urine during waking hours in a child old enough to maintain bladder control.

- It indicates involuntary loss of urine during the daytime (diurnal) after the age of five years. It can be primary (child has been persistently incontinent) or secondary if the child achieved a complete dryness for a period greater than 6 months. Urinary incontinence affects 10% of children aged 4–6 years, and 2% in adults.

- Bladder wall thickness: if greater than 5 mm, it indicates a bladder outlet obstruction such as bladder-sphincter dyssynergia in girls and posterior valve in boys.

external sphincter, often leading subsequently to increased intra-vesical pressure and kidney damage.

- In **vaginal reflux**, girls, particularly obese, who do not open their labia wide enough when voiding, urine may reflux into the vagina, then leak down and wet the knickers as they stand up.
- In boys, **posterior urethral valve** is one of the most important causes of UI. The valve is usually congenital, and if the diagnosis is missed it manifests later with recurrent UTIs, frequent urination and UI (see also Section 9.7).
- A girl who voids normally but is incontinent day and night is having an ectopic ureter with duplex kidney until prove otherwise. While an ectopic ureter in girls usually terminates within the distal third of the vaginal introitus, in boys it usually terminates within the bladder neck or posterior urethra. Therefore boys do not suffer from incontinence caused by ectopic ureter.
- Successful management of incontinence includes dietary eliminating caffeine and orange juice, improving bladder capacity by drinking extra water during daytime, treating constipation and instructing the child to void regularly every 2–3 h. Anti-cholinergic drugs are very helpful.
- Giggle incontinence occurs in about 5–10% of girls. The bladder empties completely during laughter or giggling.

It can be very embarrassing in public. Urgent management is needed.

- Daytime urinary incontinence is frequently caused or complicated by UTI. Ensure that urine is examined for UTI each time the child attends the clinic.
- When a girl presents with a history of never gaining urinary control, underwear is always wet, she probably has ectopic bladder. Confirm the diagnosis by drying the vaginal introitus and inspect the area every 15 min. Re-accumulation of urine is diagnostic.
- Treatment of a child with night and daytime wetting should focus on daytime problem first. When daytime wetting responds to the treatment, nighttime wetting will improve, not vice versa.

9.6   Polyuria

Introduction/Core Messages
- Kidney has a key role in the body water balance: an increase in plasma osmolality (even less than 1%) or decrease in blood volume stimulates osmo-receptors in the hypothalamus, leading to secretion of the anti-diuretic hormone arginine vasopressin (AVP) from the pituitary gland. AVP binds to the type 2 VAP-receptor on the distal tubules and collecting system to increase water re-absorption through cyclic AMP-mediated pathway.
- Children with polyuria (excessive urinary volume) may present with polydipsia, failure to thrive, dehydration, elevated body temperature (hyperthermia), seizure due to hypernatraemic dehydration and nocturnal enuresis.
- The most common cause of polyuria is type 1 diabetes, followed by compulsive drinking, diabetes insipidus, failure of renal tubular concentration ability (e.g. sickle cell anaemia) and renal tubular acidosis.

• Although the history and physical examination provide clues to the majority of causes of polyuria, the definite diagnosis is established from biochemical results: blood glucose, osmolality of the urine and serum, and E & U.

Differential Diagnosis

Common	Rare
Type 1 diabetes (T1D)	Sickle cell anaemia (SCA)
Psychogenic polydipsia (compulsive drinking)	Drugs (Diuretics, lithium)
Diabetes insipidus	Chronic renal failure
Renal tubular acidosis	Potassium deficiency
Hypercalcaemia	Polycystic kidney disease
	Pituitary tumours (craniopharyngioma, Histiocytosis X
	Barter's syndrome

Misdiagnosis is due to:

1st mistake: Failing to define the diagnosis of polyuria.

2nd mistake: To differentiate the main causes of polyuria: diabetes, compulsive drinking, diabetes insipidus, renal tubular acidosis and hypercalcaemia.

1. Establishing the Diagnosis of Polyuria (Table 9.7.)

2. Causes of Polyuria.
   Diabetes Type 1 (TID).

   • Of all polyuria causes, the most common and important one is T1D which is an autoimmune polygenic disease presenting with characteristic symptoms of polyuria polydipsia, weight loss.
   • Diagnosis is established by high blood glucose (HbA1c $\geq$ 6.5% or fasting BG: 7.0 mmol = 126 mg/dL). Urinalysis will confirm glycosuria and ketones in T1D.

TABLE 9.7 Diagnostic criteria of polyuria

- Polyuria is defined as urine output >6 mL/kg/h in neonates or more than 4 mL/kg/h in children resulting from either a water or solute diuresis. Polydipsia indicates water intake of >2L/m^2 or >5L/day.

- Accurate measurement of 24 h intake of fluids and quantity of urine passed should be performed to establish the diagnosis.

- Polyuria must be differentiated from a more common complaint of frequency of a small volume of urine. Mother are good historian. Observation of the child's urination helps establish the diagnosis.

- The goals of treatment are near normalisation of glucose metabolism (HbA1c < 7.5% = 58.5 mmol), and prevention of acute (hypoglycaemia, ketoacidosis) and long-term complications (retinopathy, neuropathy, nephropathy, high lipids).

Diabetes Insipidus (DI)

- DI can be central (impaired production and release of ADH from the posterior pituitary gland) or nephrogenic DI that results from resistance to the action of ADH. Table 9.8 shows the diagnostic criteria. Over 90% of cases of nephrogenic DI are caused by arginine vasopressin receptor 2 gene (AVPR2) located in chromosome 28.
- Neoplasma causing central DI presents with headaches, visual disturbances and pituitary hormonal deficiencies.
- Diagnosis is based on high plasma osmolality, hypernatraemia, and low urinary osmolality. For central DI, MRI of the pituitary may show an absence of bright signal that is considered to be pathognomonic for this type of DI. For the congenital nephrogenic DI gene identification of AVPR2 is diagnostic.

Compulsive Drinking

- Children with compulsive drinking are easily diagnosed by the long history of excessive drinking, absence of weight loss or of failure to thrive.

TABLE 9.8 Diagnosis of DI

- Clinical: DI presents with polydipsia, irritability, elevated body temperature, constipation in addition to polyuria. The preference of water over food intake results in weight loss and failure to thrive.

- Laboratory diagnosis: First morning urine: A specific gravity greater than 1.010 excludes DI. Urine osmolality >800 mOsm/kg and a serum osmolality of <270 mOsm/kg exclude DI, whereas diluted urine <300 mOsm/kg and a serum osmolality of >300 mOsm/kg confirm the diagnosis of DI.

- Water deprivation test with vasopressin can differentiate between central and nephrogenic DI.

TABLE 9.9 Diagnostic criteria of renal tubular acidosis

- RTA is characterised by defective distal acidification of the collecting tube due to genetic or acquired causes including cystinosis and drugs.

- The fourth most important cause of polyuria is renal tubular acidosis. Children may present with polyuria, dehydration, failure to thrive, anorexia and vomiting, nephrocalcinosis and renal stones.

- Diagnosis is by finding metabolic acidosis, hyperchloraemia, low serum bicarbonate and potassium, while urine's pH is alkaline (>5.5) with high urinary calcium.

- Bartter's syndrome is characterised by hypokalaemic alkalosis, hypernatraemia, hypercalciuria, dehydration and delayed growth.

- Low serum osmolality (<280 mOsm/kg) and urine specific gravity <1005 establish the diagnosis.
- Compulsive drinking needs to be differentiated from DI that has high serum osmolality and low urine osmolality (see above).

Renal Tubular Acidosis (RTA) (Table 9.9).

Hypercalcaemia

- This is defined as a total calcium >11 mg/dL (2.75 mmol/L) and due to congenital causes (e.g. Williams syndrome), or acquired causes (e.g. hypervitaminosis of vitamin D or hyperparathyroidism) or neoplasms (e.g. Lymphoma, leukaemia or neuroblastoma).

- Presenting symptoms include poor feeding, vomiting, constipation, failure to thrive, polyuria and dehydration. Polyuria due to hypercalcaemia may pass unnoticed and the infant may present in the first few weeks of life with irritability, poor feeding, weight loss, fever and seizure. These can have potentially devastation consequences (e.g. brain damage) if left undiagnosed and untreated.

- Diagnosis is established by high serum calcium. Other investigations include parathormone and vitamin levels.

9.7   Urine Retention and Failure to Pass Urine

Introduction/Core Messages

- Neurological control of the bladder consists of storage phase (stimulated by T10-L2) with sympathetic relaxation of the detrusor muscle and contracting the urethral sphincter, and voiding phase where parasympathetic stimulation facilitates detrusor muscle contraction and urethral sphincter relaxation (stimulated by S2-S4).

- Retention of urine is a frequent presentation in adults (mainly due to benign prostatic hypertrophy), but relatively infrequent in children. It is defined as inability to void for >12 h, palpable distended bladder on physical examination, or greater than expected volume in bladder in a child without previously known neurological abnormalities, voiding dysfunction, immobility or recent surgery.

- A chronically distended bladder should not be drained fully drained by catheterisation, sudden decompression can cause haematuria and other renal complications. Haematuria can cause clot in the urethra leading to urine retention and bladder distension.

Differential Diagnosis

Common	Rare
Urethral strictures, bladder neck obstruction	Bladder neck obstruction
Anuria (e.g. shock, acute renal failure)	Imperforate hymen
Neurogenic bladder	Urethral stricture
Local inflammatory (balanitis, vulvovaginitis)	Renal tubular necrosis
Dysfunction voiding (DV)	Acute genital herpes
Labial adhesion	Urethral calculus
Drugs (anticholinergic, antidepressants)	Foreign body inserted into the urethra
Urethral valve obstruction	

Misdiagnosis is due to:

1st mistake: Failing to distinguish oliguria and anuria from urine retention.

2nd mistake: Not differentiating the main causes of urine retention.

1. Characteristics of Urine Retention

   - It is important to differentiate between oliguria, anuria and retention. History, physical examination, bladder catheterisation, radiology and serum E + U distinguish the three conditions.
   - Urine retention indicates an inability to empty the bladder for >12 h with a normal or increased urine volume, or a palpable distended bladder. Causes include bladder neck or urethral obstruction.
   - Oliguria in infants is a urine output of <0.5 mL/kg/h/24 h. In older children and adults oliguria is <400/day. This quantity (usually resulting from dehydration in children) is insufficient to excrete the daily osmolar load.

- Anuria is defined as absence of any urine output. Other definition is <100 mL/day. This may result from severe dehydration or renal tubular necrosis.

2. Causes of Reduced Urine Output or Retention.
Neonates

- A healthy neonate has 6–44 mL of urine in the bladder at birth. About 90% of newborns pass urine within 24 h, the remaining pass urine within 48 h. Healthy neonates are expected to pass urine within 48 h of life, failure to void after 48 hours is abnormal and requires careful examination and investigation.
- A reduced urine output may be due to inadequate fluid intake or increased fluid loss (phototherapy or the use of radiant warmers). Other causes include circulatory failure caused by sepsis, perinatal hypoxia and respiratory distress syndrome. Renal failure can be caused by hypotension or nephrotoxic drugs.
- Posterior urethral valve (PUV) is one of the most common causes of congenital obstruction affecting the male urethra. PUV is usually diagnosed by prenatal ultrasound. If the diagnosis is not made prenatally, children later present with recurrent UTIs, poor urinary stream, urinary incontinence, frequent urination, thickened bladder wall and renal failure. Once the diagnosis is suspected prenatally, catheterisation of the bladder should not be attempted as this procedure may destroy the valve and a diagnosis can be missed.

Older Children
Labial Adhesions

- Labial adhesion or fusion of labia minora usually affects partly the posterior part of the labia and leaving a small opening anteriorly for urination. It is mainly caused by low-oestrogen in young girls. About 2% of pre-pubertal girls have this condition causing urinary outlet obstruction.
- The condition is more often asymptomatic, but sometimes girls present with dribbling incontinence or blad-

der distension. Severe adhesions can cause urine retention and renal failure.

- About 80% resolve spontaneously within 1 year of diagnosis. Some girls require topical oestrogen or surgical intervention.

Medications

- Anticholinergic drugs used to stabilise the bladder for diurnal incontinence may cause retention, dry mouth and constipation. Other medications include opioids, antidepressants and antihistamines. These cause decreased bladder detrusor muscle contractions.
- Parents should be warned about these possible side-effects.

Other Causes

Causes of urine retention in older children are numerous and include structural kidney and bladder diseases, dehydration and many infectious diseases. The details of these disorders are beyond the scope of this book.

Further Reading

Joseph C, Gattineni J. Proteinuria and haematuria in the neonate. Curr Opin Pediatr. 2016;28(2):202–8.

Mishra G, Chandrashekhar SR. Management of diabetes insipidus in children. Indian J Endocrinol Metab. 2011;15(Suppl 3):S180–7.

National Institute for Clinical Excellence (NICE). Nocturnal enuresis: the management of bedwetting in children and young people. http://guidance.nice.org.uk/CG111S.

Simmons KM, Michels AW. Type 1 diabetes: a predicable disease. World J Diabetes. 2015;6(3):380–90.

Sinha R, Raut S. Management of nocturnal enuresis-myths and facts. World J Nephrol. 2016;6(4):328–38.

Chapter 10
Genitalia/Endocrine

10.1   Precocious Puberty

Introduction/Core Messages
- Normal sexual development begins in girls with breast development, followed by the appearance of pubic hair (sometimes simultaneously with breast development), axillary hair, onset of menstruation, acne and adult body odour. In boys, it begins with testicular enlargement followed by enlargement of the penis, the appearance of pubic hair, deepening of the voice, acne and adult body odour. Puberty nowadays starts earlier than in previous generations.
- Precocious puberty (PP) is defined as puberty occurring before the age of 8 years in girls or before 9 years in boys.
- Puberty depends on increased production of a peptide (kisspeptin) in the hypothalamus resulting in increased gonadotropin-releasing hormone (GnRH), which acts on the pituitary to release the gonadotropins LH and FSH, leading to sex hormone production by the gonads.

© Springer Nature Switzerland AG 2021   205
A. S. El-Radhi, *Avoiding Misdiagnosis in Pediatric Practice*,
In Clinical Practice, https://doi.org/10.1007/978-3-030-41750-5_10

- The causes of PP are best divided into gonadotropin-dependent central (idiopathic or with identifiable causes), gonadotropin-independent (adrenal and gonadal causes) or partial PP (thelarche, adrenarche, menarche). In more than 90% of girls and 50% of boys, the cause of PP is idiopathic, i.e. no identifiable cause. The main differentiating feature between central (hypothalamic) and adrenal causes in boys is that the PP is always iso-sexual in the former and testes remain small in the latter cause.
- Full investigation such as imaging of the central nervous system and abdomen should be carried out for all children with PP who have progressive signs of puberty, are <8 years, with neurological signs or if the diagnosis is uncertain.
- Puberty can easily be assessed by bone age: if bone age is within 1 year of chronological age, puberty is either has not or just started; bone age within 2 years indicates the child is in puberty.

Differential Diagnosis (Fig. 10.1)

Common

Partial (incomplete) precocious puberty

- Premature thelarche

- Premature adrenarche

- Early menarche

Central precious puberty (e.g. idiopathic)

- Idiopathic

- CNS tumour (hamartoma)

- Irradiation of the brain

Rare

Iatrogenic external sources of sex hormone

Teratoma outside CNS (e.g. mediastinum)

Peripheral precious puberty

- Adrenal (e.g. congenital adrenal hyperplasia)

- McCune-Albright syndrome

- Ovarian tumour

Misdiagnosis is due to:

1st mistake: failing to differentiate normal variants of puberty and precocious puberty (PP).

2nd mistake: failing to differentiate partial from true (complete) precious puberty.

3rd mistake: failing to differentiate central from gonadal causes (adrenal and ovary) of PP.

4th mistake: failing to differentiate idiopathic from organic causes of PP.

1. Confirming PP

- The diagnosis of PP (signs of puberty before the age of 8 years in girls and 9 years in boys) is essential to avoid wrong diagnosis, unnecessary investigation and treatment. Significant number of children get normal variants of sexual development without true PP.

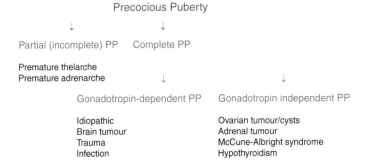

FIGURE 10.1 Short classification of PP

- Puberty is confirmed in boys by bilateral testicular enlargement (> 4ml measured by an orchidometer). Girls present with breast and pubic hair development.
- If the differentiation between normal variant of sexual development and PP remains difficult, bone age (advanced age) and pelvic ultrasound scan (pear-shaped uterus and endometrial thickness > 3 mm) suggest PP.
- Bone age in PP is advanced; hormonal levels, particularly LH, is increased.
- Lipomastia is characterised by fat deposition without glandular proliferation. It is common in overweight and obese girls who may be referred to various specialities for concern of premature thelarche. Lipomastia can be ruled out by its prominent appearance in sitting position while the breast appears much less prominent in supine position. Palpation fails to confirm firm glandular tissue. Furthermore, the inspection of the nipple and areola show no oestrogen stimulation.

2. Central (Complete, true) PP (Gonadotrophin-dependent)
   The following features favour Central PP

- Central PP is always iso-sexual arising from early hypothalamic–pituitary–gonadal activation leading to an increase of the size and activity of the gonads testes and ovaries. In girls, breast enlargement is usually the first sign of puberty; in boys it is the testicular enlargement as the first sign.
- While the nipple in premature thelarche is characteristically pale, immature, thin and transparent, in central PP the nipple is mature and prominent and dark areola indicating high circulating oestrogen.
- Causes of central PP:

    - In girls, the cause is idiopathic in >90% in girls and about 50% in boys.
    - Hypothalamic hamartoma and gliomas (e.g. neurofibromatosis) are the most common brain lesions. Careful search of the skin is essential: café-au-lait maculae have smooth border.

TABLE 10.1 Diagnostic criteria of central PP

- Boys: Increase testicular volume before the age of 9 years, followed by penis enlargement

- Girls: Development of breast, pubic hair, external genitalia and menstruation

- A bone age of >2 standard deviations above the chronological age

- LH >5 mIU/mL after GnRH stimulation test

- Low-dose radiation of the brain may induce PP in girls, high-dose may induce PP in both sexes.
- Untreated hypothyroidism.

- Early growth spurt causes rapid bone maturation, resulting in early epiphyseal fusion and short stature.
- Mental development is normal. Growth acceleration and advanced of bone age (wrist X-ray).
- Gonadotropin levels LH and FSH are increased following GnRH stimulation test.
- Table 10.1 summarises the diagnosis of central PP. MRI scan of the head is indicated particularly for boys. In girls pelvic ultrasound scan can determine the size of the uterus and pelvis.

3. Peripheral PP (Gonadotrophin-independent)

- Peripheral PP does not involve the hypothalamic–pituitary–gonad axis. It is caused by release of oestrogen or testosterone (gonadal) or from the adrenal glands.
- It can be iso- or heterosexual; the gonads are not enlarged.
- Conditions causing peripheral PP include:

  - Congenital adrenal hyperplasia (diagnosed by the signs of PP and elevated serum level of I7-hydroxyprogesterone, DHEA, cortisol and aldosterone), testicular or adrenal tumours.

- McCune-Albright syndrome (patchy skin pigmentation and fibrous dysplasia of the skeletal system, ovarian cysts, in addition of PP). The skin shows large café-au-lait patches with irregular outline that distinguish them from neurofibromatosis. Average age of PP is usually 3 years.
- Ovarian cysts and tumours are the most common cause in girls.
- Untreated hypothyroidism can cause PP; children are, however, short and the growth velocity is decreased.

- LH and TSH levels are suppressed, bone maturation is advanced.

4. Partial (Incomplete) PP

- Partial PP is either an isolated breast development (premature thelarche) or isolated pubic hair appearance (premature adrenarche) or rarely isolated vaginal bleeding (premature menarche) without other signs of puberty occurring before the age of 8 years in girls and 9 years in boys. Thelarche, adrenarche and menarche are characterised by normal growth, age-appropriate skeletal maturation, pre-pubertal uterus and ovaries and low LH and oestradiol.
- Premature thelarche is the most common cause of PP in this group, with a peak age in the first 2 years. It may be unilateral. This is usually benign, non-progressive. Onset <3 year olds is frequently associated with regression over 1–3 years, later onset usually progresses slowly to normal puberty signs. There is often increased levels of FSH, but sometimes the level is low. The condition may be caused by exogenous exposure to oestrogens. Lipomastia occurring in association with obesity should not be mistaken as premature thelarche.
- Premature adrenarche is caused by increased adrenal androgens and resulting in increased of serum

DHEA. This is also a benign condition but needs to be differentiated from conditions with androgen excess including congenital adrenal hyperplasia or ovarian tumour.

- A child with precocious thelarche or adrenarche still needs careful evaluation as these cannot be definitely differentiated from true PP. A careful history on accidental exposure or ingestion of sex hormone is important. In addition premature thelarche may progress rapidly to true PP. Therefore close observation is indicated.

5. Organic Causes of PP

- Functional causes of PP are confirmed by excluding rare organic causes.
- Brain tumours such as hamartoma are usually asymptomatic apart from PP. Therefore investigations are required to detect these lesions.
- Brain tumours that cause neurological symptoms (e.g. headaches, vomiting, cranial nerve paresis) and signs are usually malignant. Those tumours that present with PP only but without neurological manifestations are usually benign.
- Children with hypothalamic lesions often present with features such as diabetes insipidus, obesity and personal changes such as inappropriate laughing and crying.
- Causes of peripheral PP: Ovarian tumours (usually germ cell tumour) present with acute or chronic pain, abdominal distension or incidental palpable mass. Presentation of adrenal tumour is mainly virilisation (pubic hair, accelerated growth and skeletal maturation, enlarged penis or clitoris, hirsutism and acne) or with Cushing's syndrome.

10.2   Delayed Puberty

Introduction/Core Messages
- Delayed puberty (DP) is not uncommon occurring in about 2–4% of the population.
- The timing of puberty in humans is strongly influenced by genetic regulation, commonly inherited as autosomal dominant or recessive. About two-thirds of individuals with DP have a family history of late puberty.
- Current knowledge on puberty indicates that the neuropeptide kisspeptin stimulates the release of gonadotropin-releasing hormone (GnRH) from the hypothalamus to stimulate the release of FSH and LH to induce the release of the sex hormones from the gonads.
- The influence of energy supply (over- or under-nutrition) is clear. While adequate level of energy availability is required for the puberty to ensue, higher energy supply is associated with early puberty.

Differential Diagnosis

Common	Rare
Constitutional	Central nervous system tumour (craniopharyngioma)
Functional hypo-gonadotropic hypogonadism (FHH)	Hyperprolactinaemia
• Coeliac disease	Post-orchitis
• Anorexia nervosa	Prader–Willi syndrome
• Excessive exercise	Micro-penis
Structural hypo-gonadotropic hypogonadism (SHH)	Laurence–Moon–Biedl syndrome
• CNS tumour	Testicular feminisation syndrome
• Radiation/chemotherapy	Kallmann syndrome

- Pituitary hormonal deficiency

Hyper-gonadotropic hypogonadism

- Gonadal failure (Turner's, Klinefelter's syndrome)

Misdiagnosis is due to:

1st mistake: lack of definition of delayed puberty (DP).

2nd mistake: inability to differentiate the common constitutional delay from hypo-gonadotropic hypogonadism.

3rd mistake: inability to differentiate transient systemic from permanent structural hypogonadism.

1. Diagnostic Criteria for Delayed Puberty

- Delayed puberty (DP) is defined in females as a delay of pubertal changes (absence of breast bud) by 13 years or incompletion of puberty within 5 years from the occurrence of breast bud. In males, DP is defined as testes <4 mL aged >14 years, or an absence of secondary sexual signs by the age of 16 years, or incompletion of puberty within 5 years from its start.
- Puberty can be assessed by bone age (wrist X-ray): if bone age is within 1 year of child's age, puberty has not or only just started; bone age within 2 years indicates the child is in puberty.

2. Differentiating Constitutional DP from Hypo-gonadotropic Hypogonadism.

Constitutional DP

- Constitutional DP is the most common cause of DP, which is usually associated with delayed growth and positive history in the parents. In the absence of an underlying cause, constitutional DP is self-limited and benign. It is a diagnosis of exclusion and alternative diagnosis should be always considered such as hypo-gonadotropic hypogonadism (Fig. 10.2).

(Boys: testes < 4ml after 14 years of age; girls: no breast bud after 13 years of age)

↓

Family history & physical examination (excluding cryptorchidism, etc.)

↓

Exclusion: coeliac disease, CD, anorexia nervosa, IBD, excessive exercise

↓

Bone age: Boys < 13 years. Girls: < 12 years
Serum levels of FSH, LH, testosterone and oestradiol

FIGURE 10.2 Summary of steps to establish the diagnosis of DP

- Children with constitutional DP can be reassured. This is a normal variant of puberty timing with good outcome for final height and future reproductive capacity.
- While the principal cause of DP in boys is constitutional, girls have more frequent pathological causes, e.g. anorexia nervosa, chronic diseases, intensive exercise or chromosomal abnormalities.
- The bone age is delayed by over 1 year at the age of the expected puberty.
- Measurement of FSH and LH levels are increased after GnRH stimulation test.

Hypo-Gonadotropic Hypogonadism (HH)

- Hypo-gonadotropic hypogonadism is usually idiopathic due to defects in the secretion or action of gonadotropin-releasing hormone. It is characterised by low testosterone in males and low oestradiol in females in association with low FSH and LH. In contrast to the common constitutional DP, HH is a rare genetic condition.
- Functional HH occurs in coeliac disease, anorexia nervosa and inflammatory bowel disease (see below).
- Bone age is delayed over 1 year at the age of 14 years. Levels of FSH and LH remain low after GnRH stimulation test.

3. Other Causes of DP

- Turner's and Klinefelter's syndromes (discussed below).
- Girls with significant underweight and DP are likely due to anorexia nervosa or excessive sport activity, while associated obesity may suggest Prader-Willi or Laurence-Moon-Biedl-syndrome.
- Chronic diseases, e.g. Crohn's disease may present as DP, to be followed by the classical features of abdominal pain, weight loss, anaemia and high CRP level. Coeliac disease may initially manifest as DP in association with signs of malabsorption.
- Congenital micro-penis and cryptorchidism.
- Prader–Willi syndrome is a genetic disorder characterised by hypotonia, short stature, abnormal head shape, learning and behavioural difficulty, hyperphagia, later obesity and hypogonadism. The levels of human growth hormone are low.
- Laurence–Moon–Biedl syndrome is an autosomal recessive hereditary condition with polydactyly, retinitis pigmentosa (leading to gradual visual defect), obesity, learning balance difficulties.

Klinefelter's Syndrome (KS)

- KS is common occurring in one in 660 births.
- Leading symptoms and signs: tall stature (To distinguish KS form all other causes of DP) with disproportionately long arms and legs, small testes and infertility. Symmetrical gynaecomastia is common. Intelligence is usually normal but there is often a mild cognitive impairment.
- Diagnosis is confirmed with karyotyping 47 chromosome (XXY), azoospermia, low testosterone and high FSH and LH.

Turner's Syndrome (TS)

- TS (prevalence 1:2000 females) is caused by complete or partial absence of one X chromosome (X0) with characteristic features of short stature, webbed neck, cubitus valgus, lymphoedema of the hands and feet, renal (hypoplasia, aplasia, horseshoe kidney) and cardiac (especially coarctation of the aorta) abnormalities. Girls with TS have generally normal intelligence but 10% have cognitive disability. Prenatal ultrasonography may reveal findings of increased nuchal translucency, cystic hygroma or obstructive cardiac anomaly.

- Girls with TS achieve normal adrenarche and axillary hair development at appropriate age, but they do not develop menstruation.
- Karyotyping should be considered in any girl with DP and unexplained short stature. It should also be considered in females with foetal hydrops, cystic hygroma, obstructive cardiac or renal anomalies. In addition, pelvic ultrasonography and gonadotrophin estimation (FSH and LH are increased in TS) need to be considered. Growth hormone secretion is preserved in TS.

10.3   Groin Lumps/Swelling (e.g. Inguinal Hernia)

Introduction/Core Messages
- Swelling in the groin of infants and young children is common and usually noticed by the mother while giving the child a bath. Inguinal hernia (IH) and lymphnodes are the most common findings.
- Incomplete obliteration of the processus vaginalis leads to abnormal communication between the abdominal cavity and the scrotum resulting in a number of pathologies including indirect inguinal hernia, communicating hydrocele and acquired undescended testis.

- Lymphadenopathy in the groin is mostly caused by local inflammation such as nappy rash.
- Trans-illumination is used to demonstrate the presence of fluid: If light shines through, the swelling is cystic, if not the mass is solid. Ultrasonography may be required to confirm the diagnosis, particularly if an inguinal hernia is small or the child is obese, or the nature of the swelling is unknown.

Differential Diagnosis

Common	**Rare**
Inguinal hernia (IH)	Lymphatic malignancy
	Testicular feminisation syndrome
Undescended testis	
Femoral hernia	Lipoma
	Liposarcoma of the spermatic cord
	Lymphangioma
	Epididymal/epidermoid cyst

Misdiagnosis is due to:

1st mistake: failing to differentiate the main four causes of lumps in the groin.

2nd mistake: failing to establish the diagnosis of malignancy at the groin.

1. Causes of Lumps in the Groin
    Inguinal Hernia (IH)

    Diagnostic features of IH are shown in Table 10.2.

    Femoral Hernia (FH)

- FH is rare in children in comparison to IH, and characteristically appears as a soft, non-tender protrusion of abdominal contents that opens medially to the femoral vessels and below the inguinal ligament.
- Groin ultrasonography and laparoscopic examination confirm the diagnosis.

TABLE 10.2 Diagnostic features of inguinal hernia

- The history is usually diagnostic: an intermittent bulge during the day when a child is straining or crying and resolves while relaxed or asleep. Doctors confirm the swelling as non-tender and readily reducible with gentile pressure.

- Children with cystic fibrosis, undescended testes, connective tissue diseases, contra-lateral hernia and prematurity have a very high incidence of IH. Incidence in full-term infants: 1–4% (up to 30% of very low birth infants).

- In the differential diagnosis is hydrocele: both IH and hydrocele trans-illuminate, but the hydrocele does not vary in size and is not reducible on examination (see Section of Scrotal swellings).

- IH in girls is far less common than in boys. A lump in the inguinal area may contain an ovary, fallopian tube or, rarely, a testicle. The latter suggests testicular feminisation syndrome, which is confirmed by chromosomal analysis showing 46 XY. There is a high incidence of later malignancy in the gonads; it is therefore routine practice to remove them once the diagnosis is established. All girls with IH should have a pelvic ultrasound scan to exclude this syndrome.

Lymphadenopathy

- Although a child has around 600 lymphnodes, only the minority of them can be palpated in the neck, sub-mandibular, axillary and inguinal regions. Generalised lymphadenopathy involves at least two of these sites.
- Lymphadenopathy describes abnormal lymphnodes in size, consistency, and number. It can be generalised or localised.
- A normal sized lymphnode is usually < 1 cm in diameter at any site except the inguinal lymphnode which can have a size of up to 1.5 cm, and still considered normal. A size of > 2 cm may suggest malignancy such as lymphoma or granulomatous disease (e.g. TB or cat-scratch disease).
- Typical generalised lymphadenopathy occurs following Epstein-Barr infection, HIV, or systemic lupus erythematosus. Localised lymphadenopathy in the groin is mostly due to local infection such as infected nappy dermatitis.

- Malignancies in the groin include Hodgkin's lymphoma with typically present with painless lymphadenopathy with systemic symptoms such as fever, night sweats and weight loss. Rhabdomyosarcoma, a malignant tumour of the striated muscle, is the most common soft tissue sarcoma in children.

Undescended Testis

- Testicular descent occurs between 8–15 (abdominal phase) and 25–35 (inguinal-scrotal phase) weeks, gestation. Unilateral undescended testis occurs in 2–5% in full-term and in about 30% in premature babies.
- Undescended testis is defined as a testis which is neither resides nor can be manipulated into the scrotum.
- Testis in the groin occurs either because the inguinal-scrotal phase is arrested and a testis is stuck in the groin or because of ectopic testis had aberrant course of descent, e.g. pubic area (About 10% of the cases of undescended testis).
- It is important to differentiate between true undescended and the more common retractile (yo-yo) testis. The scrotum in the latter is well developed while hypoplastic in true undescended, and the testis can be manipulated down into the normal scrotal position.
- Diagnosis of undescended testis is made by unilateral empty scrotum with a palpable lump in the groin. Ultrasound is diagnostic.
- Bilateral impalpable testis with no testis elsewhere should be investigated to rule out congenital adrenal hyperplasia.

2. Malignant Mass at the Groin
   Spermatic Cord Tumours

- Rhabdomyosarcoma and lymphnode malignancy, such as lymphoma, are the most common cause of malignancy in this area.
- These tumours are rare but they are often misdiagnosed as IH. They present as unilateral hard, non-tender and immobile masses with irregular surfaces, and slowly

growing mass of the inguinal canal or scrotum. They do not trans-illuminate.

- Soft tissue sarcoma (rhabdomyosarcoma or non-rhabdomyosarcoma) in the groin presents with indolent, slowly growing tumours with non-specific or minimal symptoms. Pathological lymphadenopathy is abnormally large lymphnodes, tenderness, matted together or fixed to the skin or underlying structures, or localised in the supraclavicular area. Malignancy in this area may be associated with persistent or unexplained fever, night sweat, or anorexia or weight loss. Fine needle aspiration has a high specificity, less invasive, cheaper and quicker compared to tissue biopsy.

10.4   Penile Swelling

Introduction/Core Messages

- The foreskin is normally non-retractile and attached to the glans in neonates. It becomes retractile in about 40% of children aged 1 year, 90% aged 4 years and 99% aged 15 years.
- Inflammatory changes of the penis (e.g. balanitis and posthitis), usually with pain and redness, is the most important cause of penile swelling.
- Practically all cases of penile swelling need immediate medical attention. When a child presents with a penile problem, paediatrician has to decide whether the condition is benign and so parents can be reassured, or a prompt referral to a surgeon is needed.

Differential Diagnosis

Common	Rare
Painful swellings	
Balanitis	Lichen sclerosis
Paraphimosis	Congenital lymphoedema
Priapism	Penile torsion

Painless swellings
  Penile oedema
  Child abuse

Para-urethral cyst
Megalo-urethra
Drugs (e.g. cocaine)

Misdiagnosis is due to:

1st mistake: failing to set up characteristic features of penile inflammation.

2nd mistake: failing to differentiate the various forms of painful penile swelling.

3rd mistake: failing to differentiate the various forms of painless penile swelling.

1. Painful Penile Swelling
   Balanitis (Table 10.3)

Penile inflammation (balanitis and posthitis) is common, especially in uncircumcised boys with partly or completely non-retractile foreskin. The inflammation may be complicated by fungal and bacterial infections (candida albicans, Streptococcus spp.) and lichen sclerosis (diagnosed by the presence of a sclerotic white ring at the tip of the foreskin).

   Paraphimosis

- Phimosis is the inability to pull back the foreskin over the glans penis; paraphimosis is the inability to return it.

TABLE 10.3 Characteristics of penile inflammatory conditions

- Inflammation of the glans penis indicates balanitis while that of the foreskin is termed posthitis. Inflammation of the two penile sites indicates balanoposthitis.

- Both balanitis and posthitis are seen usually in uncircumcised children, peak age: 2–5 years of age. Balanoposthitis occurs only in uncircumcised boys.

- Balanitis, the most common cause of penile inflammation, may result from poor hygiene, allergy, seborrhoeic dermatitis, insect bites or from any erosion of the skin allowing bacteria (usually staphylococci) to invade.

- Symptoms include burning sensation, itching and pain. Signs are swelling, erythematous patches, blisters and plagues.

Paraphimosis requires immediate attention if ischaemia of the glans is to be prevented.

- Paraphimosis is commonly caused by medical professionals or parents to handle the foreskin improperly during penile examination or penile cleaning.

Priapism

- Priapism is defined as a prolonged and persistent (over 4 hours) penile erection unrelated to sexual interest or stimulation.
- Priapism is either ischaemic (with little or no cavernous arterial flow) or non-ischaemic (continuous flow of arterial blood). The ischaemic one is by far the most common type. It is typically rigid and tender. Non-tender corpora cavernous suggests the non-ischaemic type. The ischaemic type represents a medical emergency.
- Most causes of priapism are due to haematological disorders, in particular sickle cell anaemia (SCA), or glucose-6-phosphate dehydrogenase deficiency. Non-ischaemic priapism usually occurs as a result of trauma.

Penile Torsion

- A rare condition of penile swelling is penile torsion, usually anticlockwise rotation of the penis.

2. Painless Penile Swelling
   Henoch–Schönlein Purpura (HSP)

- In HSP there may be an accumulation of oedema in dependent sites that causes penile swelling.
- In addition to the penile swelling, children with HSP have characteristic purpura distribution over the extensor surfaces of the legs and buttocks, abdominal pain and arthritis. Renal involvement occurs in 20–40% of cases.

Nephrotic Syndrome

- Penile swelling may be the initial sign of the nephrotic syndrome.
- Diagnosis is established by gross proteinuria and hypoalbuminaemia.

Child Sexual Abuse (CSA)

- Physical findings due to CSA are often unrecognised, particularly in boys. Only few findings are suggestive of CSA.
- Anogenital examination should be done in all cases of alleged CSA. Findings should be documented photo- and videographically.
- The following findings may suggest CSA:

  - Acute laceration/bruising of the labia, penis, scrotum or perineum.
  - Bruising, petechiae or abrasion of the hymen.
  - Anal dilatation (in the absence of constipation or encopresis).
  - Presence of condyloma acuminata.
  - STD including gonorrhoea, chlamydia, HIV.

10.5   Scrotal/Testicular Swelling

Introduction/Core Messages
- Scrotal swelling is common in children that may be acute or chronic, painful or painless.
- The two most common painless causes are hydrocele and inguinal hernia. Hydrocele is caused by drainage of peritoneal fluid through a narrow patent processus vaginalis, while inguinal hernia is due to wide patent processus vaginalis that allows omentum or bowel to pass into the scrotum. Inguinal hernia is frequently associated with undescended testis, prematurity and connective tissue diseases such as Marfan's syndrome.
- The four most common painful causes of testicular swelling are testicular torsion, torsion of testicular appendage, incarcerated inguinal hernia and epididymitis/orchitis. These cases need urgent evaluation and surgical consultation.

Differential Diagnosis

Common

Painless swellings

- Hydrocele
- Inguinal hernia
- Idiopathic scrotal oedema
- Generalised oedema (e.g. nephrotic syndrome)
- Varicocele

Painful swellings

- Epididymitis/orchitis
- Testicular torsion
- Torsion of the spermatic cord

Rare

Testicular tumour

Trauma (scrotal haematoma)

Vasculitis

Misdiagnosis is due to

1st mistake: Failing to differentiate the main causes of painless scrotal swelling.

2nd mistake: Failing to differentiate main causes of painful scrotal swelling.

1. Painless Scrotal Swelling
   Hydrocele
     Diagnostic criteria of hydrocele are shown in Table 10.4.
   Inguinal Hernia (see Section of Groin swelling).
   Idiopathic Scrotal Oedema (ISO).

- ISO is usually caused by allergy, and may mimic scrotal torsion in presentation. The scrotum is swollen and red, but there are no other symptoms such as pain. The testis characteristically feels norma.
- The diagnosis of ISO is important to avoid unnecessary surgical exploration for suspected testicular torsion.

TABLE 10.4 Diagnostic criteria of hydrocele

- In a mobile child with hydrocele, the size characteristically increases during day time and decreases over night.

- Hydrocele is either communication (patent processus vaginalis with fluid moves from peritoneal cavity and tunica vaginalis surroundings the testis) and non-communicating hydrocele (fluid along the spermatic cord between the obliterated processus vaginalis proximally and the obliterated tunica vaginalis distally).

- Communicating hydrocele is localised in the scrotum, varies in size: minimal fluid in the morning and more fluid in the evening. The non-communicating does not change in size, usually tense and easily palpated along the spermatic cord.

- An important finding in this area is spermatic cord hydrocele, which is a fluid collection along the spermatic cord; it results from abnormal closure of the processus vaginalis and is separated from the testis and epididymis.

- It has two types: an encysted hydrocele, which does not communicate with the peritoneum, and a communicating hydrocele, where the fluid collection communicates with the peritoneum.

- Scrotal ultrasonography reveals thickening and oedema of the scrotal wall and normal appearance of the testes. Colour Doppler reveals a characteristic "Fountain Signs" which are diagnostic of this condition.

Henoch–Schönlein Purpura (HSP)/ Nephrotic Syndrome (NS).

- In HSP and NS there may be an accumulation of oedema in dependent sites that causes scrotal swelling.
- Diagnosis is clinical in HSP and confirmed by laboratory findings of proteinuria and hypoalbuminaemia in NS.

Varicocele

- Varicocele (abnormal dilatation and tortuosity of the venous plexus in the scrotum) occurs in about 15% of all adolescent boys and is a common cause of subfertility and may cause testicular atrophy. In pre-pubertal boys the incidence is <1%.
- In more severe degrees, varicocele is visible with a pathognomonic signs of "bag of worms" appearance.

2. Painful Scrotal Swelling
   Epididymitis/Orchitis

- Epididymitis is the most common cause of scrotal swelling in sexually active adolescents as part of STD. Other causes include a viral infection (e.g. mumps).
- Epididymitis/orchitis may mimic testicular torsion; the inflammation however is commonly secondary to viral infection (e.g. mumps) or STD. In addition, the scrotal swelling and pain are more gradual in epididymitis/orchitis in contrast to testicular testis. Nausea and vomiting are uncommon. The presence of fever, dysuria and pyuria suggests concomitant UTI.
- Scrotal sonography reveals hyperaemia with increased vascularisation with enlarged testis or epididymis.

Testicular Torsion/Torsion of the Spermatic Cord

- Acute scrotum is defined as scrotal pain, swelling and redness of acute onset. Venous drainage of the testis is blacked while arterial perfusion is reduced. Testicular torsion accounts for about 25% of cases.
- Prehn sign (improvement of pain when the affected testis is supported against gravity) is a useful test.
- Scrotal sonography has become a decisive tool to establish the diagnosis.

10.6 Pre-Pubertal Vaginal Discharge

Introduction/Core Messages
- Vaginal discharge (VD) is the most common gynaecological problem in children and adolescents.
- Pathological conditions of VD include non-specific vulvovaginitis (occurring in up to 70% of young girls).
- Children with VD present with pruritis, staining of the knickers, frequent urination, dysuria, enuresis, sleep disturbance due to nocturnal pruritis, or erythema of the vulva.
- Sexual abuse is a serious problem and a high index of suspicion is required to consider the diagnosis.

Differential Diagnosis

Common	Rare
Physiological	Scabies
Non-specific vulvovaginitis	Candida infection
Sexual transmitted diseases (STD)	Contact and allergic dermatitis
Foreign body	Lichen sclerosis
Threadworms	Trauma
Child abuse	

Misdiagnosis is due to:

1st mistake: failing to recognise physiological causes of vulvovaginal discharge.

2nd mistake: failing to differentiate non-specific vulvovaginitis from other more serious causes of vaginal discharge such as sexual abuse.

1. Physiological Vaginal Discharge

    - Physiologically, it occurs in neonate girls who often experience vaginal discharge (mucoid and/or bloody) as a result of withdrawal of the maternal oestrogen hormone occurring during the first two weeks of life. Any vaginal discharge after 2 weeks warrants investigation.
    - A rise of oestrogen levels at the onset of puberty causes a 2-week physiological discharge (leucorrhoea) which is milky-white or clear discharge.

2. Causes of Vulvovaginitis

    Non-Specific Common Vulvovaginitis (Table 10.5).

    Child Abuse

TABLE 10.5 Characteristics of vulvovaginitis in children

- Non-specific vulvovaginitis is the most common cause of vaginal discharge caused by poor hygiene, trauma, low local oestrogen of the vaginal mucosa, tight-fitting underwear, and the use of irritants such as bubble bath, shampoo and soaps, and close proximity of the anal orifice to the vagina allowing transfer of faecal bacteria to the vagina.

- Findings include erythema and swelling of the vulval area. The non-specific discharge is typically brown or green, has a foetid odour. Typical culture shows normal vaginal microflora or non-pathogenic bacteria.

- Pathogenic respiratory bacteria isolates are occasionally cultured and include respiratory S. pyogenes, H. influenza and S. aureus.

- Threadworm infection typically causes recurrent vulvovaginitis and manifests as nocturnal pruritis due to female worms depositing eggs on the perineum.

- Vulvovaginitis caused by candida infection is rare before puberty but may occur in infancy. Risk factors in later age include systemic use of antibiotics and steroids.

Child abuse refers to forcing children in sexual activities (penetrative or non-penetrative acts), which they do not understand or give consent to. Most perpetrators of child abuse are family close relatives or friends who typically began relating to the child during non-sexual activities to gain the child's trust. Characteristic findings are shown in Table 10.6.

Lichen Sclerosis

- Lichen sclerosis is characterised by sharply demarcated area of hypopigmentation around the vulva, major and minor labiae and the perianal area.
- It is associated with intense itching, dysuria, and bleeds easily with normal toilet activities such as genital wiping.

TABLE 10.6 Characteristic findings in children victims of child abuse

- Although clinical manifestations of child abuse may be found in the genitalia, normal physical findings of the genitalia are common, or vaginal discharge may be minimal and confused with a benign discharge.

- Vaginal mucosal injury, fresh/healed hymen damage and oral torn frenulum are important findings. Symptoms not related directly to their genitalia are common and include chronic abdominal pain, sleep disturbance, non-specific behavioural changes, school phobia, anorexia, poor school performance and social withdrawal.

- The detection of sexually transmitted disease (STD) in young children should always raise the possibility of child abuse. Therefore, screening for STD is essential. Maternal gonococcal infection causes vertical infection that manifests as neonatal purulent conjunctival and vaginal discharge after the age of 3 days of life. Neonates with syphilis present with rhinitis (snuffles), maculo-papular skin rash, hepatosplenomegaly and bone lesions. Investigation should include culture for gonorrhoea and Chlamydia, and blood for syphilis and hepatitis B serology.

Foreign Body (FB)

- Foreign body should always be thought when the discharge has foul-odour and/or blood-stained in a typical age of 3–4 years. Common objects include clumped toilet tissue or small parts of toys. Girls may insert FB either for curiosity or for sexual satisfaction.
- Complications from vaginal FB include UTI, ulceration of the vaginal walls and vesico-vaginal fistula.
- Plain X-ray, ultrasonography or MRI can establish the diagnosis. Pelvic MRI is regarded as the best tool to identify FB.

10.7   Rectal Prolapse

Introduction/Core Messages

- Rectal prolapse, RP, refers to a protrusion of the rectal wall and/or mucosa through the anus.
- The most common single cause of RP is idiopathic. Most RP have underlying predisposing causes.
- One of the most important causes of RP is cystic fibrosis (CF) and RP may be the first manifestation of the disease. CF should be considered in any case with RP.
- Most cases of RP occur during the first few years of life, but rarely in older children. In contrast to adults, incidence of RP decreases as children grow older, and conservative management is usually successful.
- RP rarely becomes chronic and chronicity is associated with complications, such as ulceration, bleeding and proctitis.
- RP has to be differentiated from rarer causes of prolapse resembling RP: prolapsed intussusception, haemorrhoids and prolapsed polyp. In addition, any child presenting with RP should be investigated for underlying causes.

Differential Diagnosis

Common predisposing factors	Rare predisposing factors
Type 1 and Type 2 RP:	Connective tissue diseases (Ehlers-Danlos)
Idiopathic	Meningomyelocele
Cystic fibrosis	Intestinal parasites
Chronic constipation	Chronic cough (e.g. Pertussis)
Chronic diarrhoea (e.g. ulcerative colitis)	Hirschsprung's disease
Malnutrition	

Misdiagnosis is due to:

1. Mistake: Failing to differentiate RP from conditions mimicking RP (e.g. prolapsing rectal polyp).
2. Mistake: Failing to consider common underlying causes of RP.

1. Differentiating RP from Conditions Mimicking RP

   - Diagnosis of RP is made by certain criteria (Table 10.7). Peak age: 1–3 years.
   - The most common cause of childhood RP is idiopathic (about 70%). Other causes such as CF should be excluded before the diagnosis of idiopathic RP is made.
   - Children with protruding intussusception are ill-looking with severe intermittent abdominal colic.
   - Prolapsed rectal polyp appears as a dark, plum-coloured, red mass in contrast to the lighter pink mucosa appearance of the RP.
   - Prolapsing polyp and hemorrhoids do not involve the entire rectal mucosa and do not have a whole in the middle.

2. Underlying Causes of RP:
   Cystic Fibrosis (CF)

   - CF is one of the most common underlying cause of RP, characterised by progressive lung disease and exocrine pancreatic insufficiency leading to gastro-intestinal malabsorption.

TABLE 10.7 Diagnostic criteria of RP

- Type 1 RP indicates the protrusion of the mucosa only, which is usually short and less than 2 cm long. It produces characteristic radial folds at the junction with the anal skin. Type 2 involves the whole thickness of the rectal wall which produces typical dark red mass.

- The diagnosis of RP is made from the history given by the parents. If rectal prolapse is present with painless, dark-red mass at the anal verge, the diagnosis is obvious. If the RP is not visible, straining or coughing by a cooperative child may produce RP. If this is not possible, parents can be requested to video-tape it when it appears. Photos and videos provide the diagnosis.

- RP is typically noted after defaecation and is reduced either spontaneously or by the child's or parent's finger.

- RP is usually painless; pain suggests complications such as ulceration, ischaemia or proctitis.

- Occult RP is diagnosed by sigmoidoscopy showing erythema and granulation of the distal rectum.

- A sweat test is indicated in all children with RP, in particular for those who present without a known underlying cause, history of cough, poor weight gain or malabsorption.

Malnutrition/Protracted Diarrhoea

- RP is more common in tropical and developing countries due to the prevalence of infective diarrhoea and parasites. Malnutrition involves the inadequate intake of calories and protein leading to impaired immunity and increased infection.

- WHO defines malnutrition as the imbalance between the intake of nutrients and energy and the body's requirement to ensure homeostasis, specific functions and growth. Acute malnutrition causes insufficient weight relative to height while chronic malnutrition causes poor height (or length) for age.

Severe Constipation (see also Constipation in Chap. 6).

- Defines as < 2 defecations/week.
- History revealed excessive straining causing increased abdominal pressure, prolonged sitting on the toilet and fiber-poor diet.
- Chronic constipation is a common cause of RP; fiber-rich diet and stool softener should help.

Connective Tissue Diseases

- Diseases associated with hypermobility/hyperextensibility of joints may develop RP.
- An important example is Ehlers-Danlos syndrome which is associated with joint hypermobility, skin fragility leading to atrophic scarring and significant skin bruising.

Further Reading

Bajpal A, Menon PSN. Contemporary issues in precious puberty. Indian Endocrinol Metab. 2011;15(Suppl 3):S172–9.

Bozzola M, Bozzola E, Montalbano C, et al. Delayed puberty versus hypogonadism: a challenge for the pediatricians. Ann Pediatr Endocrinol Metab. 2018;23(2):57–61.

Guenther P, Ruebben I. The acute scrotum in children and adolescence. Dtsch Arztebl Int. 2012;109(25):449–58.

Hernia Surge Group. International guidelines for groin hernia. Hernia. 2018;22(1):1–165.

Hobbs CJ, Osman T. Genital injuries in boys and abuse. Arch Dis Child. 2007;92(4):328–31.

Levey HR, Segal RL, Bivalacqua TJ. Management of priapism: an update for clinicians. Ther Adv Urol. 2014;6(8):230–44.

Niedzielski JK, Oszukowska E, Stowikowska-Hilczer J. Undescended testis, current trends and guidelines: a review of literature. Arch Med Sci. 2016;12(3):667–77.

Rentea RM, St Peter SD. Pediatric rectal prolapse. Clin Colon Rectal Surg. 2018;31(2):108–16. Online 2018 Feb 25. https://doi.org/10.1055/s-0037-1609025.

Stephen MD, Zage PE, Waguespack SG. Gonadotropin-dependent precious puberty: neoplastic causes. Int J Pediatr Endocrinol. 2011;2011(1):184502.

Stricker T, Novaratil F, Sennhause FH. Vulvovaginitis in pre-pubertal girls. Arch Dis Child. 2003;88:324–6.

Chapter 11
General Systemic

11.1   Excessive Crying (Baby Colic)

Introduction/Core Messages
- It is common and normal for infants to cry up to 2 h a day. When crying is inconsolable and excessive, it can cause stress to parents, disrupt parenting, and, in rare cases, place an infant at risk for abuse.
- Infantile colic is not a diagnosis; it is simply a term that describes healthy infants with paroxysmal excessive crying for no apparent reason, presumably of intestinal origin, during the first 3–4 months.
- Persistent crying beyond four months of age has been associated with long-term psychological and behavioural problems, including hyperactivity, and migraine.
- Infantile colic can be regarded as baby's way of communication. As children grow older, they find different ways to communicate.
- Although infantile colic is the most common diagnosis of excessive crying, in recent years this diagnosis is being replaced by gastroesophageal reflux (GOR).

© Springer Nature Switzerland AG 2021   235
A. S. El-Radhi, *Avoiding Misdiagnosis in Pediatric Practice*,
In Clinical Practice, https://doi.org/10.1007/978-3-030-41750-5_11

> • Colic represents a challenge to health professionals to establish the correct diagnosis of infantile colic and differentiating it from organic and non-organic conditions that may cause excessive crying. This section will attempt to provide answers to these issues.

Differential Diagnosis

Common	Rare
Colic (evening colic)	Non-accidental injury
Food intolerance (including milk intolerance)	Renal stones or gallstone
Gastro-oesophageal reflux (GOR)	Osteomyelitis
Infection (e.g. otitis media (OM))	Intestinal obstruction
Teething	Scurvy
Night terror	

Misdiagnosis is due to:

1st mistake: failing to establish the diagnosis of infantile colic: not all infantile crying is colic.

2nd mistake: failing to differentiate infantile colic from other causes of prolonged excessive crying.

1. Diagnosis of Infantile Colic

   • Infantile colic occurs in healthy infants with paroxysmal excessive crying for no apparent reason during the first 3–4 months of life. It is conventionally defined as episodes of irritability, fussing or crying for over 3 h a day, over 3 days a week and for over 3 weeks. Recently, more specific criteria for infantile colic have been proposed (Table 11.1).

   • Colic affects about 25% of infants that usually begins aged 2 weeks, peaking aged 6–8 weeks, and significantly improving by the age of 3–4 months. Attack begins suddenly, is continuous, with flushed face, tense abdomen, fisted hands and drawing up of legs.

TABLE 11.1 Rome IV criteria for infantile colic

1. Age of baby <5 m when symptoms start and stop

2. Recurrent and prolonged periods of crying, fussing or irritability that start and stop without obvious cause and cannot be prevented or resolved by caregiver

3. No evidence of failure to thrive, fever, lethargy, poor feeding or weight loss

4. Caregiver reports crying/fussing for >3 h/day or >3 days a week

5. Total daily crying is confirmed to be >3 h when measured by 24-h diary

- Colic typically is noted more in the afternoon and evening (6 p.m.–10 p.m.) suggesting that events at home (e.g. mum is busy with households; child being left alone) could be the major cause.

2. Other Causes of Prolonged Excessive Crying
   Food Intolerance (see also Chap. 6: Abdominal Pain)

- Food intolerance/allergy is a common cause of recurrent gastrointestinal symptoms in addition to the crying. The association of these symptoms differentiates it from the solitary crying of infantile colic.
- Children with cow's milk protein allergy (CMPA) and lactose intolerance (LI) usually present with symptoms of abdominal pain, flatulence and diarrhoea occurring within 30–60 of ingestion milk. In addition, LI is associated with perianal skin irritation and excoriation. Stool faecal pH is low <5.5.
- A positive family history of atopic disorders (eczema, wheezing, food allergy) supports the diagnosis.
- Improvement of symptoms after eliminating the suspected food item and substituting it with extensively hydrolysed or amino acid-based formula (in case of CMPA) or after excluding lactose (in case of LI) for two weeks supports the diagnosis.

- Skin prick test and serum-specific IgE can help in the diagnostic evaluation in CMPA. Detection of reducing sugars and low pH in stool, and positive breath hydrogen testing confirm the diagnosis in LI.

Gastro-Oesophageal Reflux (GOR)

- GOR is considered physiological when there is posseting/vomiting only. This occurs in 40–65% in otherwise healthy infants between the ages of 1 and 4 months.
- When GOR is causing complications (e.g. inadequate weight gain, excessive crying, irritability, disrupted sleep, gagging or choking during or at the end of feeding, apnoea and/or poor weight gain), it is termed GOR disease.
- Other less common but important presentations include dystonic posture (Sandifer's syndrome) and respiratory symptoms (e.g. wheezing, recurrent pneumonias).
- Both conditions, cow's milk protein allergy and GOR, are commonly coexist in both infants and children.

Infection

- Infection such as otitis media can cause prolonged crying.
- Associated features, such as fever, pulling the ear, preceded viral upper respiratory tract infection, point towards the correct diagnosis.

Non-Accidental Injury

- Clinicians should be aware of the possibility of non-accidental injury for unexplained baby crying. The presence of inadequate baby's weight and bruises in the skin should provide clues for the diagnosis.
- Early increase in crying in a healthy infant is the most common stimulus for shaken baby syndrome (abusive head trauma). This is a potentially lethal form of physical abuse causing brain injury, e.g. subdural haematoma, with 80% significant brain injury and 20% deaths.

Pain and Crying Associated with Teething

- The question as to whether teeth eruption causes further symptoms is controversial. In the past, serious diseases were attributed to teething. Hippocrates thought that teething caused itching gums, fever, convulsions and diarrhoea. In 1842, teething was the registered cause of death in 4.8% of all infants who died in London under the age of one year and 7.3% of those between the age of one and three years.
- Nowadays, while some still believe that teething produces nothing but teeth, others believe, as the majority of mothers do, that it is associated with increased body temperature. There is no strong evidence to support claims of systemic signs, including fever, at the time of teeth eruption. The time of tooth eruption may be associated with increased salivation and irritability in children.

11.2   Excessive Weight Gain (Obesity)

Introduction/Core Messages
- Obesity is a very common and a serious problem in children. Its incidence has increased dramatically since 1970, and this rate is likely to continue. Children with special needs are at increased risk of obesity.
- Childhood obesity is linked to adult obesity with the potential risk of increased mortality, cardiovascular disease, hypertension, diabetes, back pain, hyperlipidaemia, cholelithiasis and sleep apnoea.
- Obese children often do not eat more than their peers. Genetic factors and reduced energy output (long hours sitting in the front of TV and computer) are more important causal factors.

- A common reason for seeking medical help for child's obesity is parental concern whether the 'child's glands' are normal. Obesity usually has no 'glands' as an underlying cause.
- Obesity is usually the result from increase in the number of the fat cells (adipocytes) occurring during gestational months and during the first year of life.
- Although growth hormone (GH) is not increased in simple obesity, obese children tend to have increased leptin level, protein binding and insulin-like growth factor 1 (IGF-1).
- There are currently no drugs available that can be recommended for use in children.
- A definition of obesity often lacks precision, and other causes of obesity are not considered. Although hormonal and endocrine causes of obesity are rare in clinical practice, it is essential to consider them in the differential diagnosis of an unexplained obesity. These issues will be discussed in this section.

Differential Diagnosis

Common	Rare
Simple obesity	Endocrine (e.g. Cushing's disease)
Infant of diabetic mother	Genetic syndromes (e.g. Turner's syndrome)
Drugs (e.g. steroids, pizotifen, anticonvulsants)	Beckwith–Wiedemann syndrome
Polycystic ovary syndrome (POS)	Insulinoma
	Cerebral gigantism (Sotos syndrome)
	Laurence–Moon–Biedl syndrome

Misdiagnosis is due to:

1st mistake: failing to establish the diagnosis of simple nutritional obesity.

2nd mistake: failing to differentiate simple obesity from other causes of secondary obesity such as endocrine, syndromes and POS.

1. Confirming Simple Nutritional Obesity

- Simple obesity is characterised by abnormal or excessive fat accumulation (adiposity) that increases risk to health. Diagnosis is only confirmed when weight measurements are carried out.
- Because of the social stigmata, overweight and obese children are vulnerable to discrimination, low self-esteem and depression.
- In children up to 24 months, the diagnosis of overweight and obesity is based on the weight-to-length ratio. After the age of 2 years, it is based on the body mass index (BMI) (Table 11.2).
- The main cause of childhood-onset obesity is not over-eating, but genetic (usually confirmed by a detailed family history) and decreased energy output. The latter can be estimated indirectly by the total hours spent in the front of TV and computer per day.
- In contrast to obese children due to endocrine causes, children with simple obesity have accelerated linear growth and are usually taller than non-obese children.

TABLE 11.2 Diagnostic criteria of overweight and obesity

Age	0–2 years	2–5 years	5–18 years
Index	Weight-to-length ratio	BMI	BMI
>85th centile	At risk of overweight	At risk of overweight	Obese
>97th centile	Overweight	Overweight	Obese
>99th centile	Obese	Obese	Severe obese

However they are not tall as adults and their final height depends on the genetic potential of growth.

2. Characteristics of Secondary Obesity (Endocrine and Syndrome Obesity)

The following features favour secondary obesity:

- Early onset of obesity <5 years with rapid progression.
- Rapid weight gain in association with reduced height velocity or short stature.
- Delayed cognitive development.
- Dysmorphic feature.
- Ocular and /or auditory abnormalities.
- Cryptorchidism or hypogonadism.
- Use of drugs that may cause hyperphagia, e.g. corticosteroids, sodium valproate.

3. Endocrine Causes of Obesity

Cushing Syndrome (CS)

- CS is caused by exposure of excess glucocorticosteroids largely from the pituitary gland.
- Children with CS are differentiated from those with simple obesity by being short, have delayed bone age and delayed onset of secondary sexual characteristics.
- Clinical features include facial plethora and truncal obesity with thin limbs. Fat distribution in simple obesity is diffuse. Striae in simple obesity are pink, occurring after rapid growth in adolescents, while these marks appear earlier in Cushing syndrome and are violaceous.
- Blood pressure is high in children with CS (also elevated in simple obesity sooner or later).
- Diagnosis is established by confirmation of increased cortisol (serum cortisol levels, 24 h urine collection). MRI scan for the pituitary and ultrasound scan are required.

Polycystic Ovary Syndrome (POS)

- POS is the most common endocrine disorder in reproductive aged women occurring in 5–15%.

- Clinical and/or biochemical evidence of androgen excess (hyperandrogenism) causing menstrual disturbances, overweight and hirsutism and deepening voice.
- Evidence of oligo-ovulation or anovulation.
- Ultrasonic evidence of polycystic ovary.
- The syndrome is often associated with insulin-resistant hyperinsulinism and acanthosis nigricans (hyperpigmented area which may also be associated with internal malignancy), and type II diabetes.

Pseudo-Hypoparathyroidism

- This condition is characterised by resistance to the action of the parathyroid hormone.
- Clinical features include blunting of the 4th and 5th knuckles of the hand in association with hypocalcaemia (causing carpopedal muscular spasm) and high phosphate.

4. Obesity Associated with Syndromes
   Cerebral Gigantism (Sotos Syndrome)

This is a genetic overgrowth disorder (incidence 1:14,000) that manifests as:

- Excessive rapid overgrowth (prenatal overgrowth) with height and weight >97th centile.
- Characteristic facial features with acromegalic appearance and prominent forehead.
- Increased head circumference (>97th centile) with advanced bone age.
- Early intellectual disability with behavioural autistic problems.
- The majority of cases have genetic mutation on the NSD1 gene.

Prader–Willi Syndrome

- Associated features include infantile hypotonia with poor sucking and poor feeding, hypogonadism, typical facial appearance (narrow bifrontal diameter, short nose) and mood instability.
- Children later develop hyperphagia that leads to obesity.

Laurence–Moon–Biedl Syndrome

- This is an autosomal recessive genetic disorder with different gene mutations (BSS gene).
- Clinical features include obesity, visual defects (rod-cone dystrophy), moon face, short stature, polydactyly, male hypogonadism, diabetes, renal dysfunction and developmental delay.

Beckwith–Wiedemann Syndrome

- This is an overgrowth disorder characterised by abdominal wall defect (exomphalos, umbilical hernia), gigantism (height and weight >97th centile) and visceromegaly (e.g. macroglossia, cardiomegaly), and anterior ear lobe creases.
- Other clinical features include hemihypertrophy, embryonal tumour, renal abnormalities and diffuse adrenal glands, and tendency for hypoglycaemia. This condition predisposes to tumour formation such as Wilms tumour and hepatoblastoma.
- There is chromosomal alteration on chromosome 11p15 (molecular testing).

11.3   Failure to Thrive and Unexplained Weight Loss

Introduction/Core Messages
- Growth is based on food intake, its metabolism, gastrointestinal absorption and psychosocial factors.
- Failure to thrive (FTT) is a descriptive term, not a diagnosis, with a peak incidence occurring in children 1–2 years of age. FFT is divided into two main categories: organic and non-organic causes. Globally, malnutrition/under-nutrition is the most common cause of FTT.

- If the history and physical examination do not suggest a specific underlying organic disease such as malabsorption, psychosocial causes are likely in high income countries, and laboratory and imaging are unlikely to provide the answer.
- In FTT, weight is the first centile affected, followed by length if the FTT persists; head circumference (HC) is only affected if FTT is prolonged.
- Early recognition of FTT is essential because it leads to growth reduction and cognitive and behavioural problems.
- Diagnostic errors occur when a diagnosis of FTT is made without considering normal growth variants (1st mistake). In addition, although there is agreement that organic causes must be excluded in cases of FTT, they are often not considered or difficult to differentiate from non-organic causes (2nd mistake).

Differential Diagnosis

Common	Rare
Psychosocial (e.g. emotional deprivation, neglect)	Malignancy
Eating disorder (e.g. anorexia nervosa)	Severe gastro-intestinal reflux
Milk allergy	Inborn error of metabolism
Malabsorption (e.g. coeliac disease)	Inflammatory bowel diseases
Malnutrition and under-nutrition (from poverty)	Chronic diseases
Chronic infection (e.g. HIV, parasitic)	Induced illness (Munchausen by proxy)

Misdiagnosis is due to:

1st mistake: wrongly diagnosing those children with normal physiological variations as cases of FTT.

2nd mistake: failing to establish diagnostic criteria of FTT.

3rd mistake: failing to differentiate between non-organic and organic causes of FTT.

1. Normal Growth Variants

   The following normal growth variants should be considered before diagnosing FTT:

   - Prematurity. A misdiagnosis commonly occurs if the weight is uncorrected for gestation. These children have appropriate weight for height and growth velocity.
   - Intrauterine growth retardation (IUGR) often leads postnatally to small-for-date, which is defined as <10th centile for gestational age. If the IUGR originates from the first trimester, it usually affects the weight, height and head circumference (HC), and is termed symmetrical IUGR, Those cases of IUGR that originate from the 3rd trimester produce asymmetric IUGR.
   - Catch-down growth. Some babies with large weight (e.g. infants of diabetic mothers) decrease their birth centile by major centiles over their next 6–18 m to lower centile curves to match their genetic potential. They continue to grow along their new centile curve. They should have normal development and physical examination.
   - Familial/genetic short stature. Infants born to small parents are typically small from birth, and grow along their low centile for both weight and height. These children reach their adult height (based on mid-parental height) according to their genetic potential. Their bone age correlates with their chronological age, unlike those children with constitutional growth delay (see next).
   - Constitutional growth delay (CGD). This is a normal variation of growth characterised by normal size at birth, prolonged prepubertal growth but a normal growth velocity. During the immediate pre-pubertal growth, the growth slows down considerably. Puberty is delayed but occurs eventually at a normal sequence. The hallmarks of CGD is delayed bone age.

TABLE 11.3 Diagnostic criteria of FTT

- Weight < 2nd centile weight gain on growth chart, with decreased velocity of weight gain that is disproportionate to height

- Weight decrease of 2 or more major centile lines

- Delay weight gain is significantly less than expected for their age

- A single measurement showing weight centile is markedly disproportionally from height and head circumference

2. Diagnostic Criteria of FTT

- Although there is no agreement about a definition of failure to thrive (FTT), a child whose weight is below the 2nd centile or more accurately below 0.4 percentile on the 9 percentile chart is a case of FTT as shown in Table 11.3.
- Generally, FTT is caused by inadequate intake of nutrients required for growth, nutrient malabsorption that prevents the bioavailability of ingested nutrients, or increased metabolic demand due to a chronic, genetic or metabolic disorder.

3. Differentiating Non-Organic from Organic FTT
   Non-Organic FTT (NOFTT)

- NOFTT (also referred to as psychosocial NOFTT) is far more common than organic causes. It is due to inadequate or insufficient intake of nutrition either because of economic factors or parental neglect with no apparent growth-inhibiting organic disease.
- Medical history is diagnostic when it includes birth history, family medical history, parental occupation and income, marital and employment status, and nursery or school attendances. Normal findings on physical examination support the diagnosis.
- Neglect, either nutritional or emotional, is the most common cause of underweight in infancy, accounting for more than 50% of cases of NOFTT. Children at high

risk of this type of abuse are those with excessive crying in infancy, physical handicap, chronic illness and those with behavioural or learning difficulty.

- Early detection of psychosocial problems (e.g. neglect) is very important because it can result not only in poor physical growth but also in poor cognitive and intellectual development.
- Depression disorder is not uncommon in adolescents who may show either a decrease or increase in weight.

Organic FTT (access to sufficient nutrition)

This is an uncommon cause of FTT occurring around 20% of cases.

Eating Disorder

- Weight loss in adolescent girls is likely to be due to eating disorder. Diagnosis can be difficult in early stage.
- Asking about attitude toward eating and weight will suggest the diagnosis.

Malabsorption (see also Chap. 6: Abdomen).

- Malabsorption is characterised by diarrhoea of >4 stools a day and/or steatorrhoea, that is fat content in stool >4 g a day for infant, and >6 to 8 g in older children. The most common cause is coeliac disease.
- Coeliac disease is an important cause of malabsorption with specific human leukocyte antigen (HLA-DQ2 and HLA-DQ8) Symptoms are characterised by irritability, diarrhoea, weight loss and anaemia.

Pancreatic Insufficiency

- Exocrine pancreatic insufficiency is defined as a reduction of the pancreatic enzymes to a level that is inadequate to maintain normal digestive function.
- Pancreatic insufficiency results from pancreatic disorders, e.g. cystic fibrosis (CF), chronic pancreatitis or resection. Typical features of exocrine insufficiency include bloating, abdominal pain, diarrhoea, steatorrhoea, weight loss. Low level of vitamin D may lead to

osteoporosis and low level of vitamin A may lead to visual impairment.

- Shwachman–Diamond syndrome is an autosomal recessive disorder and is the second most common cause of pancreatic insufficiency after CF. In addition, the syndrome is associated with neutropenia due to bone marrow failure, and skeletal abnormalities.
- Diagnosis of exocrine pancreatic insufficiency depends on the cause. Stool pancreatic elastase is diagnostic.

Short Gut Syndrome (SGS)

- SGS is defined as a clinical condition that results from surgical resection, congenital defect or disease-associated loss of absorption leading to inability to main nutrient balance when fed with a normal diet. These clinical conditions include volvulus, gastroschisis, aganglionosis, intestinal atresia, necrotising enterocolitis.
- SGS usually requires prolonged parenteral nutrition due to intestinal failure.

Inflammatory Bowel Diseases (IBD)

- IBD, including ulcerative colitis (UC) and Crohn's disease (CD), are increasing in incidence in paediatric population. Classical presentation includes weight loss, abdominal pain and diarrhoea (bloody in UC). Other symptoms are poor growth, and extra-intestinal signs (erythema nodosum, arthritis, autoimmune hepatitis).
- Laboratory data include anaemia, thrombocytosis and hypoalbuminaemia. Low stool calprotectin makes IBD unlikely and differentiates it from IBS.

Prader–Willi Syndrome (PWS)

- PWS is a complex neuro-behavioural condition mostly (70-75%) due to deletion in the paternally inherited chromosome 15q11-q13 region.
- Children with PWS have two nutritional stages: initial poor feeding and poor weight gain in infancy in association with hypotonia, followed by hyperphagia that leads to obesity in older children.

Chronic Infections

- Chronic infections include lung, liver, pancreas, kidneys and helminthic infections.
- HIV infection (initially called in Africa "the slim disease") causes FTT because of abnormal gastrointestinal absorption and inadequate psychosocial support.

Metabolic Disorders

- These include renal tubular acidosis, lactase and sucrase deficiency, hereditary fructose intolerance.
- Associated features include vomiting, hypotonicity, lethargy, seizures.

Other Organic Causes of FTT
These include cleft lip and palate, swallowing incoordination, milk and food allergy.

11.4   Tiredness/Fatigue

Introduction/Core Messages
- Everyone experiences fatigue, but recovery is rapid following a rest or a good sleep.
- Most childhood diseases, particularly infections, cause fatigue, which may last for many days and sometimes weeks.
- Chronic fatigue syndrome (CFS), also known as myalgia encephalomyelitis, is diagnosed after taking a careful history, recognition of the pattern of symptoms and the exclusion of other illnesses causing fatigue.
- There is little knowledge about diagnostic criteria of CFS. More importantly, there are numerous conditions that present with prolonged fatigue which are confused with CFS.

Differential Diagnosis

Common	**Rare**
Chronic fatigue syndrome (CFS)	Malnutrition/chronic anaemia
Post-viral fatigue	Obstructive sleep apnoea
Cancer-related fatigue	Hypokalaemia
Autoimmune diseases	
Depression	
Neuromuscular diseases (e.g. Myasthenia gravis)	
Adrenal insufficiency	
Fibromyalgia	
Drugs (e.g. anti-histamine)	

Misdiagnosis is due to:

1st mistake: Not adhering to the diagnostic criteria to define CFS.

2nd mistake: Failing to differentiate CFS from other causes of prolonged fatigue.

1. Chronic Fatigue Syndrome

CFS is defined as an unexplained, persistent and overwhelming tiredness, weakness or exhaustion causing disruption of daily life and resulting in a decrease of physical and/or mental work, unrelieved by sleep. The condition typically exacerbates by exercise or physical activity. A minimum of 3 months is required before diagnosis is made. CFS is rare before the age of 10 years. Sometimes it follows an infection, e.g. EB-virus. The diagnosis is established by history and the exclusion of other fatiguing diseases (see below). Girls are more commonly affected than boys.

Diagnosis is based by obtaining a careful history, recognition of the pattern of symptoms and exclusion other conditions that might explain the symptoms. Characteristic clinical diagnostic features are summarised:

Primary Symptoms

- Unexplained fatigue that persists for days and weeks without relief by rest and sleep, and worsens following minimal physical or mental activity.
- Prolong post-exertional malaise that increases after physical, mental and emotional exercise.
- No restoration of energy after sleep, in addition to difficulty in initiating and/ or maintaining sleep.
- Condition results in substantial reduction in previous levels of occupational, educational, social activities.
- Symptoms are unexplained by other condition.

Secondary Symptoms (most symptoms should be present)

- Impaired cognitive function and concentration.
- Myalgia, multiple-joint arthralgia but no swelling or redness.
- Sensitivity to sound and light.
- Sore throat (non-exudative pharyngitis).
- Tender cervical or axillary lymphnodes.
- Laboratory tests are usually normal and are performed to exclude other conditions mimicking CFS.

2. Differential Diagnosis of CFS (Table 11.4)
   Post-Viral Fatigue

- Post-viral fatigue has a short duration of illness compared to those of CFS.
- A history of a viral infection at onset and laboratory evidence support the diagnosis of post-viral.
- Post-viral fatigue is less debilitating compared to patients with CFS.

Depression

- Depression is a serious disorder that has increased in recent years among children and adults.
- Diagnosis is made by the criteria in the Diagnostic and Statistical Manual of Mental Disorders (DSM-lV).

TABLE 11.4 Conditions to be excluded from CFS

Post-viral fatigue	SLE
Adrenal insufficiency	Narcolepsy
Depression	Obstructive sleep apnea
Depression .	Cancer-related fatigue
Myasthenia gravis	Auto-immune diseases
Fibromyalgia	Medications
Chiari malformation	

- Comorbidities are common and include anxiety, obesity, posttraumatic stress disorder, chronic diseases. Child abuse is a major contributory factor.

Cancer-Related Fatigue

- Is defined as a distressing, persistent with physical, emotional and cognitive tiredness or exhaustion related to cancer or its treatment that is not proportional to recent activity.
- Fatigue is debilitating and most common and distressing side-effect of cancer treatment, occurring in 30–60% of cases.
- Diagnosis is established by symptoms arising from the site of the cancer and the history of treatment.

Autoimmune Diseases

- Autoimmune disease are chronic conditions initiated by loss of immunological tolerance to self-antigens and mediated by B-cells and T-cells. They are common affecting 5–10 of population. Females are predominately affected. The exact cause is unknown.
- Autoimmune diseases have diverse clinical manifestations but children commonly present with fatigue, low-grade fever and poor concentration. Juvenile idiopathic

arthritis, SLE and juvenile dermatomyositis are examples of autoimmune diseases (see Arthritis section for detail).

- Diagnosis is related to the specific disease of the group. Screening tests include antinuclear antibody (ANA), auto-antibody, immunoglobulins, CRP and ESR.

Myasthenia Gravis (MG)

- MG is an autoimmune antibodies-mediated disorder involving the neuromuscular synaptic transmission and causing fluctuating fatigability/weakness of the skeletal muscles.
- Characteristic features include ocular muscle involvement causing ptosis, and bulbar muscle weakness causing fatigable chewing, and weakness of other proximal limb muscles.
- The fatigue is characteristically worse after repetitive activity and improves after rest. Fatigability is worse late in the day.
- Diagnosis is established by IV Tensilon (Edrophonium) test, while the patient is observed for improved muscle strength.

Adrenal Insufficiency (Addison's disease = AD)

- Presentation is with symptoms of fatigue/weakness, failure to thrive, weight loss syncope, abdominal pain and depressive mood.
- Diagnosis of AD is established by the presence of hypotension, hypoglycaemia, hyponatraemia, hyperkalaemia and hyperpigmentation of the skin and mucous membranes. Corticosteroid stimulation test confirms low cortisol level after 30–60 min. Other tests include auto-antibodies, CT scan of the abdomen to image the adrenal glands, and MRI for the pituitary gland.

Fibromyalgia

This is characterised by:

- Widespread non-inflammatory musculoskeletal pain/ aches at 3 or more sites with 5 or more of 18 typical tender points for ≥3 months.
- Minor criteria include fatigue, poor sleep and co-morbid anxiety. In contrast to CFS, fatigue is not prominent.
- Absence of an underlying condition such as injury or inflammatory process.
- Normal laboratory tests.

Medications
Many drugs can cause fatigue such as anticonvulsants and antihistamine.

11.5 Unexplained Persistent Fever (UPF)

Introduction/Core Messages
- When the history and physical examination fail to identify a specific source of fever in an acutely ill, nontoxic-appearing child, usually aged 3–36 months, the illness is termed 'fever without localized signs or fever without a focus = FWF'. About 20% of all febrile episodes demonstrate no source of infection on presentation. The most common cause is a viral infection, mostly occurring during the first few years of life. Such an infection should be considered only after exclusion of urinary tract infection (UTI) and bacteraemia. Unexplained persistent fever comprises FWF and pyrexia of unknown origin (PUO).
- FWF is defined as an acute and persistent febrile illness without apparent source that lasts for less than a week, with the history and physical examination not capable to find the cause. PUO is defined as fever without localising signs that persists for over 1 week during which evaluation fails to detect the cause.

- In PUO, infections are the most common causes, accounting for 60–70% of all cases, of which about 15% of are due to viral infection. Collagen diseases account for about 20%, of which the most common cause is juvenile idiopathic arthritis (JIA) as a pre-arthritic presentation. Malignancy presenting as fever without other manifestations may occur in up to 5%. Miscellaneous diagnoses account for 5–10% and undiagnosed in the remaining 5%.
- Other causes include non-JIA collages/vascular diseases, drugs, allergy, and periodic fevers.

Differential Diagnosis

Common	Rare
Viral infection (e.g. human herpes-6 (HH-6))	Inflammatory bowel disease
Urinary tract infection (UTI)	Neoplasms
Occult bacteraemia	Drug fever
Collagen diseases (e.g. JIA, SLE)	Periodic or relapsing fever
Parasitic infections (e.g. Malaria, Lyme disease)	Subacute thyroiditis (de Quervain's disease)
	Apical tooth abscess
	Occult abscess
	Anhidrotic ectodermal

Misdiagnosis is due to:

1st mistake: having little and basic knowledge about fever

2nd mistake: failing to approach systematically the causes of unexplained persistent fever.

3rd mistake: failing to differentiate non-infectious from infectious causes the fever.

4th mistake: failing to differentiate bacterial from viral infections.

1. Basic Knowledge About Fever

    Fever (pyrexia) may be defined in both patho-physiological and clinical terms:

    Patho-physiologically, fever is an interleukin-1 (IL-1) mediated elevation of the thermoregulatory set-point of the hypothalamic centre. In response to an upward displacement of the set-point, an active process occurs in order to reach the new set-point. This is accomplished physiologically by minimising heat loss with vasoconstriction and by producing heat with shivering. Behavioural means of raising body temperature include seeking a warmer environment, adding more clothing, curling up in bed and drinking warm liquids.

    Clinically, fever is a body temperature of 1 °C (1.8 °F) or greater above the mean at the site of temperature recording. For example, the range of body temperature at the axilla is 34.7–37.4 °C, with a mean of 36.4 °C; 1 °C above the mean is 37.4 °C. The following degrees of temperature are accepted as fever.

Rectal temperature	≥38.0 °C
Oral temperature	≥37.6 °C
Axillary temperature	≥37.4 °C
Tympanic membrane	≥37.6 °C

    Fever is also defined as a core temperature of 38.3 °C or higher, i.e. just above the upper limit of a normal body temperature.

    The importance of at least 1 °C higher than the mean temperature lies in the diurnal variation of normal body temperature, which reaches its highest level in late afternoon (4–6 pm) and lowest prior to awakening (4–5 am).

2. Causes of UPF (Unexplained Persistent Fever)

    Important diagnostic clues:

- The history should be searched for animal exposure, travel abroad and prior use of antibiotics.
- Repeated physical examinations are more helpful in establishing a diagnosis of FWF and PUO than extensive investigations.

- Physical examination begins by observing the child's appearance (e.g. ill-looking), alertness, quality of cry, degree of playfulness and response to stimulation.
- Eye examination looking in particular for uveitis as an early clue for rheumatoid arthritis, bulbar conjunctivitis for leptospirosis, choroid tubercles and toxoplasmosis lesions.
- Noting that an absence of sweat with high fever may suggest heat stroke, dehydration, anhidrotic ectodermal dysplasia or familial dysautonomia.
- A child with the initial diagnosis of FWF or PUO on presentation to the hospital may often prove to have either a self-limiting benign disorder, such as viral infection, or a common disease that can be diagnosed easily with simple initial investigations, such as urine culture or a chest X-ray. Therefore, provided that the child's condition is satisfactory, extensive investigations initially are not required. An atypical presentation of a common disease is more common than a rare and exotic disease.
- Causes of unexplained persistent fever that lasts < 1 week (FWF) and > 1 week (PUO) are shown in Tables 11.5 and 11.6, respectively.

3. Differentiating Non-Infectious from Infectious Fever:

- Differentiating infectious from non-infectious causes of fever is crucial. Clinicians consider the presence of fever to be generally caused by an infection and therefore non-infectious causes are rarely thought to be the cause. Table 11.7 shows features that support the presence of non-infectious and infectious causes of fever. Main causes of fever.
- Infections: Bacterial, viral, TB, parasitic and rickettsia are by far the most common cause of fever in children. Infection remains the likely diagnosis in a febrile child until proven otherwise.
- Non-Infectious: collagen/vascular, malignancy, drugs, allergy, recent immunisation, periodic fevers.

TABLE 11.5 Main causes of fever without a focus of infection (FWF}

Causes	Examples	Clues for diagnosis
Infection	Bacteraemia/ sepsis	Ill looking, high CRP, leukocytosis
	Most viruses (HH-6)	Well appearing, normal CRP, WBC
	UTI	Urine dipsticks
	Malaria	In malarial or being in malarial area
Collagen	JIA	Pre-articular, rash, splenomegaly,
	High ANF, CRP	
Drug fever	Most drugs	History of drug intake, diagnosis of exclusion

HH6 human herpes-6, *UTI* urinary tract infection, *ANF* antinuclear factor, *CRP* C-reactive protein, *JIA* juvenile idiopathic arthritis

TABLE 11.6 Principal causes of PUO

Cause	Reason for being a case of PUO
Infection (60–70%)	
Localised	
Sinusitis	standard sinus imaging not performed or negative
Endocarditis	previously unsuspected of having a cardiac defect
Occult abscess	absence of clinical signs
Systemic	
Viral (e.g. EBV)	fever as the only sign, no organ involvement
TB	extrapulmonary, tuberculin test negative

(continued)

TABLE 11.6 (continued)

Cause	Reason for being a case of PUO
Kawasaki disease	incomplete presentation, diagnosis not considered
Brucellosis	diagnostic tests for Brucella not performed
Collagen (about 20%)	
JIA	pre-arthritic manifestation
SLE	atypical manifestations
Neoplasms (5%)	
Leukaemia, lymphoma	atypical presentation; unusual localisation, blood tests negative
Neuroblastoma	disseminated
Miscellaneous (5–10%)	
Drug fever	diagnosis not considered, suspected drug not stopped
Factitious fever	diagnosis not considered, thermometer left to patient
Auto-inflammatory disease	Absence diagnostic criteria

4. Differentiating Viral from Bacterial Infections

- Viral infections, affecting mainly the upper respiratory tract (URT), are the causes of fever in about 90–95%% of febrile children. It is the physician's primary role to identify the remaining 5–10% of children who have a bacterial infection and who may require antibiotic treatment. Children with viral infection will usually require only symptomatic treatment. With stomatitis, varicella or other readily identified exanthems, the

TABLE 11.7 Features suggestive of non-infectious and infectious causes of fever

Features in support of non-infectious causes of fever

- History (e.g. recent vaccination, drug intake)

- Physical examination and laboratory tests failed to detect an infection

- Low-grade fever, absence of chills and diurnal rhythm of fever

- Associated pruritic rash, multiple joint involvement

- Negative cultures (blood, urine, stool, CSF)

- Fever not responding to antibiotics but to steroids

- Absence of leukocytosis and left shift, presence of antinuclear factor (ANF)

Features in support of infectious causes of fever:

- Underlying conditions, e.g. immunocompromised status, splenectomy, sickle cell anaemia, neonates and young infants, presence of intravascular catheters

- Fever >39.0 °C or greater, presence of chills, diurnal fluctuation of fever

- A focus for infection (e.g. tonsillitis, pneumonia)

- Rapid response of fever to antibiotics in bacterial infections

- Leukocytosis >20,000 in bacterial and leukopenia <500 in viral infections

- High procalcitonin (PCT), CRP levels

cause of the fever is apparent, and further diagnostic evaluation may not be required.

- Patients with impaired immune status including those on chemotherapy, sickle anaemia cell disease, human immunodeficiency virus infection or cystic fibrosis should be considered to have a bacterial infection until proved otherwise.

- Often it is difficult to differentiate viral from bacterial infections based on clinical features alone but on combining these features with laboratory means (Table 11.8).

TABLE 11.8 Differential diagnosis of viral and bacterial infections

Diagnosis of a viral infection as a cause of fever is supported by:

- Viral infections are the main causes of fever in 90–95% of all febrile children

- Involvement of several organs at the same time (e.g. URTI)

- History of nursery attendance or being in contact with people with similar symptoms

- Well-appearing, playfulness and interacts well with his parents

- Normal CRP, PCT and leukocytes. Presence of leukopenia, lymphocytosis

- Positive detection of viral antigens with enzyme immunoassay (ELA), fluorescent antibody (FA) or electron microscopy

Diagnosis of a bacterial infection as a cause of fever is supported by:

- Localisation of the infection to one organ (e.g. ears or tonsils)

- High fever (>39 °C), duration (>3 days) and the presence of rigor

- Pre-existing disorders, e.g. immunosuppression, splenectomy, sickle cell anaemia

- Irritability, lethargy, ill-looking with a weak cry and who is uninterested in the surroundings

TABLE 11.8 (continued)

- Laboratory findings:

    - WBC >15000 (Neonates more often have leukopenia of <5000–10,000)

    - CRP: >10 (neonates); >40 (older child)

    - Procalcitonin: >0.5ng/mL

    - CSF: >8 WBC/mm^3

    - Urine: positive nitrate on dipsticks, urinalysis showing >10 wbc/hpf

    - Chest radiograph: infiltrate

    - Stool: >5 wbc/hpf stool smear

Further Reading

Berger AM, Mooney K, Alvarez-Perez A, et al. Cancer-related fatigue, version 2:2015. J Natl Compr Cancer Netw. 2015;13(8):1012–39.

Daelemans S, Peeters L, Hauser B, et al. Recent advances in understanding and managing infantile colic. Version 1. F1000Res. 2018;7:1426. https://doi.org/10.12688/f1000research.14940.1.

Dahlen HG, Foster JP, Psalia K, et al. Gastro-oesophageal reflux: a mixed methods study of infants admitted to hospital in the first 12 months following birth in NSW. BMC Pediatr. 2018;18:30.

El-Radhi AS. Physical treatment of fever. Arch Dis Child. 2000;83:369.

El-Radhi AS. Clinical manual of fever in children. Cham: Springer Verlag; 2017.

Nutzenadel W. Failure to thrive in children. Dtsch Arztebl Int. 2011;108(38):642–9.

Rowe PC, Underhill RA, Friedman KJ, et al. Myalgic encephalomyelitis/chronic fatigue syndrome diagnosis and management in young people: a primer. Front Pediatr. 2017;5:121.

Valerio G, Maffeis C, Saggese G, et al. Diagnosis, treatment and prevention of pediatric obesity: consensus position statement of the Italian Society for Pediatric Endocrinology and Diabetology and the Italian Society of Pediatrics. Ital J Pediatr. 2018;44:88.

Index

© Springer Nature Switzerland AG 2021   265
A. S. El-Radhi, *Avoiding Misdiagnosis in Pediatric Practice*,
In Clinical Practice, https://doi.org/10.1007/978-3-030-41750-5

Printed in the United States
By Bookmasters